Praise for *Called Again*

"What an outstanding read! Not only is it an excellent chronicle of an extraordinary accomplishment but, at its essence, it is a love story—love for hiking, love for the trail, and love for a spouse. In remarkably readable prose, Pharr-Davis shares insights into her life and her spirit, which are at once inspiring and humbling. Over the course of her 46-day journey, Pharr-Davis encounters hardship, revelation, and insight all while continuing to deepen her love for all that is most important in her life. It is, quite simply, a transcendent story and one that I wholeheartedly recommend!"

> — Andy Jones-Wilkins, Ultra-Runner, Educator,
> and ten-time Western States 100-miler Finisher

"*Called Again* is reminiscent of the trail itself. The story completely absorbs you and carries you along with a patient but relentless rhythm, urging you forward to devour page after page. Called Again is also simultaneously, complete not about the trail or the record, it is about reaching inside yourself to discover who you really are. Yes, this book inspired me to want to discover the AT and my limits on the trails, but more importantly, it inspired me to continue to relentlessly pursue the person I am meant to become."

> — Devon Yanko, a two time National Champion
> in the 50 mile and 100k distance and a
> 2012 Olympic Trails Marathon Participant.

"Jennifer Pharr Davis is one of the most competitive and mentally tough people that I have met in my 43 years of coaching. It is no surprise that she's accomplished all that she set out to do on the trail and in her personal life. What I love about her books—*Becoming Odyssa* and now *Called Again*—is that I learn a lot about her and even more about myself."

> — Don Meyer, one of college basketball's all-time
> winningest coaches, recipient of the 2009 Jimmy V
> Espy Award for Perseverance and 2010 Naismith
> Basketball Hall of Fame's Lifetime Achievement Award

"As a professional athlete, I can't imagine walking forty-seven miles a day for forty-six consecutive days! What an incredible challenge, both physically and mentally. Jennifer accomplished a truly remarkable feat and has an amazing story to tell."

— Josh Willingham, Major League Baseball player since 2004 and winner of a 2012 Silver Slugger Award with the Minnesota Twins

"Beauty is an action as much as an aesthetic. This is the story of Jennifer Pharr Davis and her husband Brew working together to accomplish something beautiful—and something most people thought was impossible. Their hard work, faith, and love for each other are inspiring."

— Andie MacDowell, Actress

"[The] writing is a reverberating catalyst for readers' reflections into their own choices of abilities, freedoms and dependencies."

— Eustace Conway, subject of Elizabeth Gilbert's *The Last American Man* and star of *Mountain Men* on The History Channel

"Called Again is a refreshingly personal and absorbing story. Jennifer Pharr Davis is clear-sighted in her understanding and her relationships with others. She uses language with such skill that an ordinary hiker can appreciate both the beauty of the trail and its challenges."

— Chuck McGrady, National Sierra Club President 1998-2001

CALLED

AGAIN

CALLED

AGAIN

A STORY
of LOVE
AND
TRIUMPH

·

JENNIFER

PHARR DAVIS

BEAUFORT
BOOKS

Library of Congress Cataloging-in-Publication Data

Davis, Jennifer Pharr.
Called again : a story of love and triumph / by Jennifer Pharr Davis.—
First edition.
pages cm
ISBN 978-0-8253-0693-8 (hardcover : alk. paper)—
ISBN 978-0-8253-0745-4 (pbk. : alk. paper)—
ISBN 978-0-8253-0653-2 (ebook)
1. Davis, Jennifer Pharr. 2. Hikers—United States—Biography. I. Title.
GV199.92.D37A3 2013
796.51092—dc23
[B]
2013002077

For inquiries about volume orders, please contact:

Beaufort Books
27 West 20th Street, Suite 1102
New York, NY 10011
sales@beaufortbooks.com

Published in the United States by Beaufort Books
www.beaufortbooks.com

Distributed by Midpoint Trade Books
www.midpointtrade.com

Printed in the United States of America

Interior design by Elyse Strongin, Neuwirth and Associates, Inc.
Interior illustrations by James Pharr
Cover image by code6/E+/getty images
Design by Oliver Munday
Lyrics from Mumford and Sons

First to Him,
Next to him,
And then, these four women:
Mom, Maureen, Meredith and Margot.

HEARTACHE

JULY 2007

When I was twenty-four years old, I learned that heartache is consuming. There was a pain in my chest, my body felt weak, and my bottom eyelids were a tired dam trying to hold back a river of tears.

In June 2007, I was stuck in the thick, shoe-sucking mud of my own disappointment. I was ankle deep in despair, and I couldn't move forward. The only thing that came easily was sleep. I retreated to that liberating darkness as often as I could. When I was forced to leave my bed and face the world, I struggled to keep my lips from trembling. My fake grin was like a small Band-Aid placed on a wound that was much too large to conceal.

I had lost my first love.

It didn't make sense to me. We had found each other on the Appalachian Trail, and we had shared hundreds of miles that melded us together like the seam-seal glue on our backpacking gear. Over the past two years, we had hiked to the highest point in the lower forty-eight states, we had forded rivers with torrents of water that rose past our waists, we had crossed snowfields where only our ice axes prevented us from sliding to our deaths. If we could overcome all that, why couldn't we overcome ourselves?

In the midst of this pain, the only thing I wanted to do was return to the trail. The trail provided me with a purpose. It was a catharsis and it provided a way to move forward physically, even if my heart was held captive. And if miles were the best medicine, then I wanted to hike as far and as fast as possible.

I needed guidance. I emailed the legendary hiker Warren Doyle for advice.

> *Warren,*
>
> *I can't believe where the trail has taken me since attending your Appalachian Trail Institute in 2004! It was great to see you briefly last summer on the Pacific Crest Trail. I don't know if you heard, but I finished the 2,633-miles in late September. I have been able to thru-hike some other, shorter trails, and now I want to try a new challenge. This summer, I want to go back to the Appalachian Trail and try to see how fast I can hike it. I think that I could set the women's record. I know you set a trail record in the 1970s. Do you have any suggestions for me?*
>
> *Thanks so much!*
>
> *Jen*

Warren quickly replied:

Jen,

Trail records are about endurance, not speed. If you are interested in doing an endurance record, you should try for a record on a shorter trail and see if you like it before attempting it on a trail that is over 2,000 miles long. Are you currently in Virginia? I am traveling up I—81 this evening. We can meet at the gas station on your exit and have a planning session. I should be there at 12:30 AM.

Warren

Just before midnight, I started driving toward the interstate. I struggled to keep my eyes open. I knew from my previous interactions with Warren that his internal clock was different from most people's. I respected that, but I couldn't really relate to it. All my body had wanted to do for the past few weeks was sleep—especially in the middle of the night.

When I arrived at the gas station, Warren was already there waiting for me. We each bought a large coffee and then sat down at a table to talk.

"Why do you want to try a trail record?" he asked.

Ugh, Warren and his questions! They were never about gear, or logistics, or a schedule. The first thing he always wanted to know was *why*. I knew I had to make it through this test before he would talk to me about hiking specifics. But how could this sixty-year-old man understand a twenty-four-year-old woman's broken heart?

I sighed deeply, staring at the steam rising from my coffee, then I began. "Well, I love thru-hiking, and now I've hiked over 6,000 miles on my own. So I want to try something different. Plus, I'm having a tough time right now, and I think going back to the trail and trying for a record would be healing."

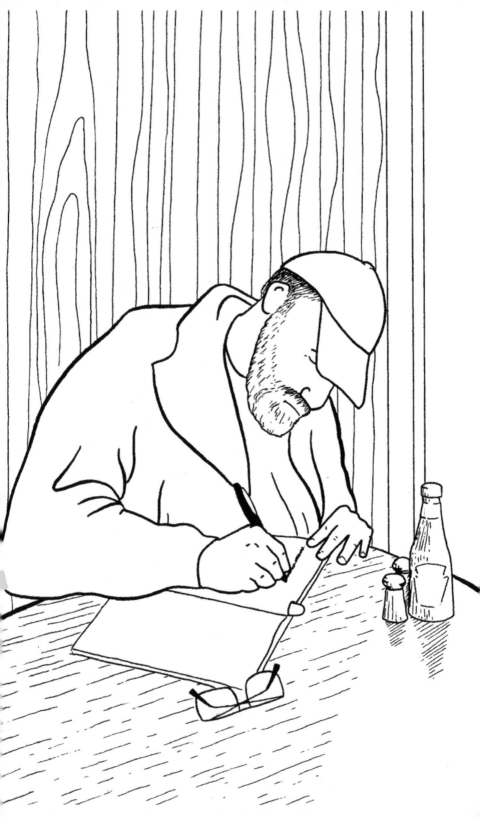

"Healing?" Warren scoffed. "You think physically hurting and reaching new levels of discomfort is going to be healing?"

The inquisition had begun.

"Well, yeah," I replied. "Emotionally, I have a lot of weight right now, and I know that the trail has a way of stripping off the excess layers of worry, fear, and even pain. I was hoping that a record attempt would help me get to a better place faster."

I looked up at Warren, expecting to see a frustrated sage trying to deal with a young woman's melodrama. But when I caught his eye, I saw a friendly glimmer and a knowing smile on his face.

"So this is really a conversation about lightweight backpacking?"

"Well, yeah, I mean, most of my gear is lightweight," I replied.

"No, not your gear —your heart."

Warren spent the next hour telling me about how the trail had helped him through different joyous and painful milestones in his life. The trail helped him process his college graduation, the birth of his children, a divorce from his first wife, and a new marriage. He explained that every time he visited it, he was a new person, and even after forty years and over a dozen completions of it, he was still learning from each new day he spent out there.

After he helped me understand the healing and reflective role that the Appalachian Trail had played in his life, Warren then looked me in the eyes and told me I should consider the Long Trail.

The Long Trail is a two-hundred-seventy-two-mile footpath that runs the length of Vermont. It is the oldest long-distance trail in the country, and it contains some of the most tedious and difficult hiking terrain. I had heard enough about the Long Trail to know that it was composed more of roots and rocks than dirt. It contained numerous exposed summits that seemed to attract high winds and violent lightning storms, and some sections of forest were so dense that not even the sun could penetrate the trees. Plus, the remote northern portion of the trail was isolated to the point that one simple mistake could have huge consequences. It sounded like it might be just what I needed.

Warren took out a twenty-year-old guidebook and helped me plan an eight-day itinerary for the trail. Finally, I had a plan and a schedule. But before I could leave, Warren had one more thing to teach me.

As we exited the gas station and headed to our cars, Warren turned to me and asked, "Do you know how to waltz?"

"Waltz?!" I repeated. "I thought you were here to help me walk, not waltz."

"They're very similar," he replied.

Warren put a tape in the cassette player of his rusted old car and turned up the volume. He walked over to me and bowed. Then, with the grace of an eighteenth-century English gentleman, he stretched out his hand. I put my fingers in his palm, and together, at three o'clock in the morning, we danced in the dark parking lot of a gas station off Interstate 81.

My feet occasionally stumbled or stepped on Warren's toes, even though I looked down and tried to will them in the right direction. But Warren softly instructed, "Look up. Listen to the melody. If you want to dance, then you can't fight the music; you have to flow with it."

2

THE LONG TRAIL

AUGUST 2007

One of the thru-hikers who finished the Appalachian Trail with me broke my heart; the other helped to mend it.

On my way to Vermont, I stopped in Connecticut to see Mooch. After my first hike on the Appalachian Trail, I hadn't expected to stay in such close contact with him (or to continue dating Nightwalker). But our experience had been so intense and our bond so unique that we couldn't figure out how to move on without one another. Like me, Mooch had sworn off thru-hiking at the top of Katahdin. And like me, he had spent every summer since on a long-distance trail. In fact, he had completed the Long Trail just a few weeks prior to my visit.

After ten hours of driving, I pulled into a driveway in Trumbull, Connecticut. Mooch was sitting on the steps to his apartment. I was disappointed to see that he no longer had the long, curly hiker-hair or shaggy beard that he sported on the trail.

As soon as I stepped out of the car, he walked over to me and engulfed me in his long, lean arms. He whispered into my ear, "Oh, Odyssa. Sweet, sweet Odyssa. It's so good to see you." He paused. "But you are a *mess*! You're going through heartbreak, not a thru-hike. You know you *can* still take showers, right?"

My friend laughed, grinning from ear to ear. I smiled too. I was pleased to see that Mooch still had the same kind spirit and offensive sense of humor that had made even the worst situations on the trail seem tolerable.

Next, he lowered his nose to my synthetic tank-top and inhaled near the crook of my neck. "You know, dressing—and smelling—like you do on the trail isn't going to bring Nightwalker back. Come on, Odyssa. Let's get you inside and under a showerhead."

I heard what Mooch was saying, and I appreciated the unique way that he was able to console my aching heart with criticism, but in that moment all I could think about was how nice it was to hear the name Odyssa. I missed trail names and the personas people took on when hiking. Odyssa embodied strength and adventure, the ability to overcome adversity. I felt that if Odyssa could overcome the challenges of the hike, if she could find a way to traverse the Long Trail in eight days, then Jen could somehow overcome her broken heart.

That afternoon, after a much-needed shower, I sat in Mooch's apartment going through my pack and separating my food into zipper-lock bags while Mooch sat on his couch humming and strumming his guitar.

"So you really think you can finish the trail in eight days?" he asked indignantly.

"Yeah, if things go well."

"Odyssa, you know it took me three and a half weeks to hike the Long Trail, and I was going at a solid pace. The northern half is as difficult as the Appalachian Trail in Maine and New Hampshire." Then, prodding me, he continued, "I don't think you can do it."

I looked up at Mooch and saw a smile reaching almost to the bottom of his ears. He knew me well enough to know that being told I couldn't do something was the best motivation I could receive.

The next morning, after cooking me a large hiker breakfast of eggs, pancakes, and bacon, Mooch drove me to the Vermont-Massachusetts border and the southern terminus of the Long Trail. When we arrived at the trailhead, the last thing I wanted to do was get out of my friend's air-conditioned car and step into the late-summer heat wave. I should not have hesitated. It was like looking off a bridge before BASE jumping.

Suddenly, none of this made sense. How was hiking a difficult trail with an impossible goal going to solve anything? I didn't want to face my problems or the trail. All I wanted was to go back home, back to my bed, and sleep.

Mooch looked over at me, reading the doubt in my eyes, and quickly responded, "Oh no you don't."

He got out of the car, removed my pack from the trunk, and then walked around to the passenger door. In a last-ditch effort, I tried to push the lock button, but it was too late. Mooch lifted the outside handle and the warm blanket of humidity wrapped around my body.

My friend reached in and grabbed my elbow to help me out of the car. "Remember, this is what you wanted," he said. "Plus, I like to see you suffer. So c'mon, out we go."

With a little more pulling and prodding, I climbed out. Mooch hoisted my green backpack—filled with gear and several days' worth of food—onto my shoulders. I tightened the straps around my chest and the buckles around my waist and gave Mooch one last long, wistful hug. Then, just like the day before, he whispered softly in my ear, "It's time. Let go."

So I did. I let go and started slowly up the hard-packed dirt trail littered with worn gray rocks and surrounded by verdant outstretched arms of mountain laurel. Within seconds, the thick green tunnel hid Mooch, and I was on my own.

I took one step after another. My breathing fell into a rhythm, and after hiking a mile, all of the anxiety that I had experienced at the car vanished. I felt better than I had in weeks. I felt at home.

My euphoric return to the trail lasted all of seventeen hours. After leaving Mooch and camping at the border, I began my trek the next morning at six a.m. and hiked forty-six miles that day. Forty-six miles! It was the farthest that I had ever traveled by foot in a twenty-four-hour period.

During the morning, I felt light and the miles passed quickly. By the afternoon, my legs started to stiffen and my pace decreased. And as the daylight turned to dusk, my shoulders ached, my hips were sore from my pack weight, and the lower half of my body cried out with pain and fatigue. My skin was cold to the touch and my stomach was empty. Even my brain felt tired. As simple as walking was, it was hard to focus on putting one foot in front of the other for sixteen straight hours.

But I didn't feel completely horrible because my chest felt warm and full. I was proud of coming so far in such a short amount of time. I had made it to the north side of Stratton Mountain, and now the disappearing sun and my exhausted legs told me it was time to find a camping spot.

As the forest faded into darkness, I continued to walk, searching for a flat spot to lie down. But I was not paying attention to the path in front of me, and as a result, I stepped on a large, loose rock. The stone rolled out from under me, and my left leg twisted as I fell.

My first response was to get up as quickly as possible. I never liked to assess injuries sitting down because things always seemed worse from the ground perspective. If I could self-diagnose while standing or walking, then the prognosis was never as bleak. I put most of my weight on my hands and unfolded my lower limb as if I were trying to come out of a difficult yoga pose. Then I transitioned back to a Homo erectus stance. My knee was sore but steady, and everything seemed to be okay. I took a few more steps to rebuild my confidence and loosen my knee, then I found a place where the shoulder of the trail was wide. I unrolled the light foam pad and unpacked my thin down sleeping bag.

I crawled inside my bed and took a brief moment to look up at the stars. It was a very comforting scene. The twinkling lights were far more magical and hopeful than the pale white ceiling of my bedroom.

When I awoke the next morning, I knew even before I sat up that my left knee was *not* okay. It felt hot and stiff, and I was barely able to contort it to get out of my narrow sleeping bag.

When my kneecap came into view, it was swollen and pink. I poked at the bulging flesh with my finger. It now looked and felt like a serious injury, and based on previous ailments that I had incurred on the trail, I realized that there was only one cure: I had to keep hiking.

While doctors recommend rest, ice, compression, and elevation, I knew that increased circulation, a large range of motion,
and gritted teeth had fixed many of my trail injuries in the past.
The pain might increase before my knee felt better, but that was
part of the healing process.

I reached for my shoes and carefully placed my left foot into the
sneaker, but something inside didn't feel right. I figured it must
be from the altered state of my knee, and I reached for my other
shoe. Then I noticed something orange underneath the tongue. I
looked closer and spotted a pinky-sized slug adhered to it.

"Uck." I picked off the slug and hurled it onto a nearby tree. Then
I reached into the toe-bed and found two more slimy creatures.
Chills went down my spine as I unlatched them and flung them
into the woods. I was not scared of slugs, but I didn't care to handle
them, especially first thing in the morning. I put my shoe on and
started to stand up when an unpleasant thought crossed my mind.

"Nooo!" I took off my other shoe, and just as I had suspected,
my sock was completely covered in opaque orange goo. Judging
from the high concentration of gunk, there had been at least as
many slugs in my left shoe as in my right—and none of them had
survived.

That morning was miserable. Every other step hurt, and walking
on uneven terrain intensified the pain. During a treacherous descent down a boulder field, I placed my hands on two neighboring
rocks to brace my step, and as I eased my foot down into a small
crevice, I felt something bite my ankle. I looked down and saw
a large yellow jacket. Suddenly, I was overcome with adrenaline,
and I ran the next forty yards down the trail.

I have a moderate allergy to bees, and the thought of my throat
swelling shut trounced the pain of my aching knee. Once I was a

safe distance away, I looked down and saw two red bull's-eyes. I immediately took some Benadryl and put my EpiPen in my hip pocket in case I started wheezing. The ache in my knee returned, now accompanied by a sharp pain in my ankle. I kept hobbling down the trail and watched my shin change shades of red and then swell until it resembled a doughnut just above my low-cut sock.

For the rest of the day, I was not focused on a trail record. I was only focused on putting one foot in front of the other. I didn't care how slowly I hiked. I just wanted to keep moving forward. As the sky grew dark, I came to a cold creek where I submerged both of my legs. The muscle definition in my left leg was gone. It was red and swollen from my toes to my lower thigh, and it was hard to look at, let alone bend.

After completing two and a half days and over a hundred miles on the Long Trail, my leg was still inflamed, I was still in pain, and I was coming to a road. Few long-distance hikers would quit their treks if it were not for the constant presence of roads. Roads are a reminder of creature comforts, food, and social support. Physically and emotionally, roads are the most dangerous place on the trail.

As I approached U.S. 4, every part of my body was yelling at me to abandon the hike. I was willing my feet down the north slope of Killington, listening for the roar of the highway and contemplating what to do, when I heard an adult voice singing "The Itsy Bitsy Spider." It was an appropriate serenade considering how many spiderwebs I had hiked through that morning, but where was it coming from? I turned down a switchback and saw a grown man jogging up the trail with a toddler on his shoulders. Both the man and the little boy smiled and said hello as they passed me, and they continued to sing as they turned up the next switchback.

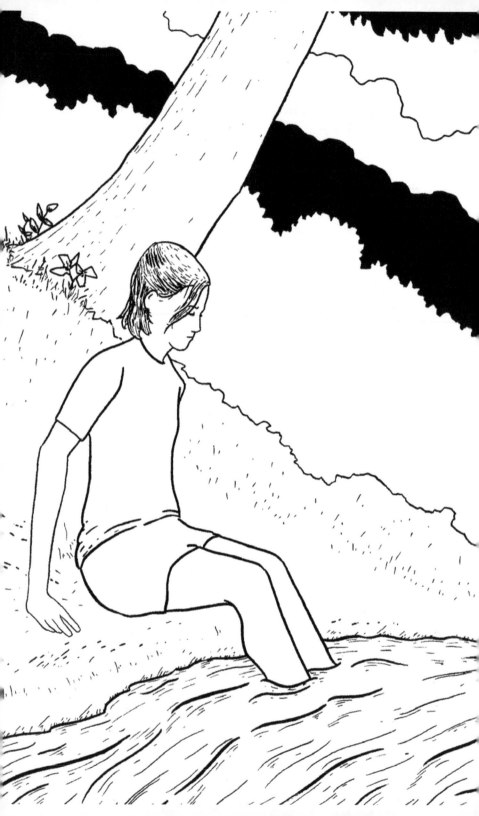

At first, I was frustrated by the encounter. I was having trouble walking downhill, and this man was happily pacing uphill with a sixteen-month-old on his shoulders—while singing! But despite my bitterness, there was something too innocent and joyful about the encounter for me to stay sour. In fact, in a strange way, I felt attracted to the man—or at least to what he represented.

I thought about my ex-boyfriend and my broken heart. As miserable as the pain in my left leg had been, it was all consuming. And that had been a blessing. But now, after passing the father and son on the trail, something inside me felt hopeful. I had been part of a great relationship with a great guy who loved life, loved me, and loved the trail. But there were other great guys out there. Guys who would run up a trail with their child on their shoulders, singing corny kid songs. That was my type of guy.

As I spotted my first car through the trees, I no longer wanted to quit. And just as I exited the woods, I heard a voice calling from behind me.

"Hey! Hey, wait up. Are you a thru-hiker?" It was the father and son bounding back down the mountain. And I could tell just by the way the man said "thru-hiker" that he either was one or wanted to be one.

"I'm thru-hiking the Long Trail," I replied. The first hundred miles follow the same path as the Appalachian Trail, so I wanted to differentiate my 272-mile journey from the 2,180-mile one.

"That's awesome," he said, smiling. "My wife and I thru-hiked the A.T. for our honeymoon several years ago." *I knew it.* "We're up here vacationing with our kids. Do you need any trail magic?"

I thought about that question. The first time someone offered me trail magic, I had been hesitant to accept because as a society we are taught not to accept gifts from strangers. But now I loved getting help from people I didn't know. It was one of my favorite parts of the trail.

At this point, however, I didn't need any food or a ride into town. I looked down at my red, irritated leg. It was covered in lacerations from a thorny section of overgrown trail, and they were starting to ooze puss. If I didn't clean them out soon, there was a good chance they would get infected.

Finally, I responded. "Well, I could really use a shower."

"Great! We're staying just a few miles down the road. You can shower at our place."

Within the span of an hour, I went to their rental cabin, met the man's equally gracious thru-hiker wife and their three-year-old daughter, showered, cleaned my leg, iced my knee and ankle, and administered anti-inflammatory pills and salve. I also ate a large portion of homemade vegetable lasagna and then returned to the trail.

Back at the trailhead, the mom and dad stood at their car, attaching babycarriers for a second afternoon hike. The kids were yelling and looking for the orange slugs I had told them about. As I continued hiking into the woods and away from Vermont Route 4, my body didn't hurt as much, and neither did my heart.

Putting my life back together started at the base of Pico Peak that day. I no longer thought about quitting the hike. Instead, I pushed onward each day with the goal of reaching Canada as quickly as the trail would permit. Unfortunately, the path was not overly permissive.

Once the Long Trail split from the A.T., I traveled through several patches of overgrown stinging nettles. The invisible hairs that hung from the leaves of the plant quickly attached to my legs and caused a burning sensation that lasted anywhere from five to fifteen minutes. At times, the pain was so intense that I could only manage by screaming at the top of my lungs until it subsided.

The trail was all but deserted in central Vermont, and I doubt anyone ever heard me yell, but if they did, they probably dialed 911 out of concern.

The weather on the second half of the hike was as bad as it could be in the summertime. In every twenty-four-hour period, it rained for at least eighteen hours. More often than not, the downpour was accompanied by lightning and thunder.

The water turned the mountain slopes into a treacherous minefield of slick stones and boulders. During the lightning storms, I felt less threatened in the dense hardwood forest, but I was often delayed near the summits where there was no protection. Sometimes I hid underneath rock outcroppings and inside trail shelters, waiting for the storms to pass. Over and over again I would count the seconds between the lightning and thunder, hoping that the storm would weaken, but it seemed locked in place.

The heavy rain reminded me of the countless tears I had shed over the summer. So in the midst of hiking through the storm, I talked to God. It was not a prayer of reverence or thanksgiving. Instead, I complained and literally cried out to God, blaming him for my broken heart. I asked over and over why my last relationship didn't work out and what I was supposed to do now. I wanted an immediate answer, but all I got was more thunder and lightning.

The trail threw one punch after another: bad weather, slick rocks, poorly marked junctions, and just when I thought I had covered the most difficult stretch, I came to Doll Peak. The elevation of the mountain did not compare to the unending slope of Mount Mansfield, the highest summit on the Long Trail. And the climb was not as technical as the boulder scramble near Camel's Hump in central Vermont. But for my tired, sore, soaking-wet body, this felt like the toughest ascent of the trail.

When the trail becomes technical, you are frequently forced to place your hands on boulders or trees to gain balance. Sometimes you have to attach your hiking poles to your pack and use arm strength to pull yourself up a steep pitch. Technical trail can also demand sitting and sliding or crab walking down a mountain. If nothing else, the degree of difficulty increases since every step could result in a sprained ankle or twisted knee.

As I hiked up Doll Peak in the pouring rain, I used both hands to scramble and maintain my balance. I spent enormous energy willing my thighs in front of my body, then hoping my calves and feet would follow. With every step I tried to put my shoes on large, stable-looking rocks to prevent a fall. But it didn't work.

I fell five times in five minutes. My legs weren't going where my mind told them to, and on top of that, I couldn't see the next few yards through the clouds and fog, let alone the summit. I wanted to sit down and give up. But that wasn't an option, not in this weather and not on this terrain.

Just then, I remembered something Warren had said when we were waltzing at the gas station near I-81 in the early morning hours. "You can't fight the music, you have to flow with it."

There I was in the middle of a nor'easter, my knee was swollen, and scrapes and bruises covered my body, but I was still out there in the terrible, awesome onslaught of the wilderness. And I knew that I had to keep pressing forward. I realized that all summer I had been hiding from my own soundtrack. I hadn't wanted to hear the music; I'd just wanted to sleep and cry, to reject the truth that was blaring all around me.

Warren was right. I needed to embrace the rhythm, not worry so much about falling. And right now, the storm was my music and the rocks were my dance floor. So as I continued up the trail, my chin lifted and my footsteps grew stronger and more certain.

When I made it to the top of Doll Peak, I let out a victory cry. I wanted it to sound tough, but instead it sounded like a squeaky cheer at a pep rally. For me, those cries never seemed to reflect the guttural emotion that had formed them. Nevertheless, I was deeply proud to be on the top of that barren mountain in the Northeast Kingdom of Vermont, that physical and emotional barrier that I had overcome—and I only fell twice on my way back down.

After seven days, fifteen hours, and forty minutes, I reached the Canadian border. I had danced the dance, I had felt the pain, and now I could hear the music changing. The rain had stopped and so had my tears.

I felt lighter than I had in months. The Long Trail had allowed me to express my sadness and my frustration. It had allowed me to scream and cry; it had given me an arena to hurt. And I learned that sometimes the hurt has to get worse before it can get better.

By the end of the trail, I also felt that God had given me an answer through all my yelling and pleading. The first time I thru-hiked, it was to figure out who I was and what I was going to do with my life. But it wasn't until this trip that I finally realized the trail was more than a solitary adventure or something to check off my bucket list. The trail was my passion, and now I wanted it to be my profession.

I had big plans. I couldn't wait to call Warren and tell him about my hiking adventure and my new resolution. The next day, as soon as I had cell service, I dialed his number.

"Hello?" he answered.

"Warren, it's Jen."

"What's wrong?" he asked.

"Nothing's wrong. I'm done with the trail."

"You're already finished?" Warren asked in disbelief.

"Yep. I finished in less than eight days. That's good enough for the record, isn't it?"

"Yes, it certainly is."

"Well, it was awesome," I said excitedly. "I can't wait to tell you all about it. And I think I figured a lot out while I was hiking. I will be driving home in a few days, so maybe I can stop by and fill you in on everything."

"I would love that," Warren replied. "What you accomplished is just incredible."

"Thanks, Warren. Oh, hey, I was wondering . . . who had the unsupported record on the Long Trail before me?"

Warren chuckled. "Well, until this morning, I did."

After our phone call I felt shocked and a little embarrassed. I should have been able to figure out on my own that Warren held the previous record. After all, he could never have given me such good advice if he hadn't been there before.

On my drive home, I started making plans for my new hiking company. I wanted to help other people get outdoors. I was convinced that the trail was the best and the cheapest therapy I knew. By taking other people into the woods, I hoped that they could experience some of the joy, serenity, and truth that I felt in the wilderness. Plus, I knew that personally, I wanted—no, I needed—to keep hiking. Now that I had set a record on the Long Trail, my attention was focused on the Appalachian Trail.

Warren was right to suggest a shorter trail for my first record attempt, but now that I had gotten a taste, I wanted the full course dinner. A record attempt was more focused and more difficult than a traditional thru-hike. It required discipline and intensity, and it stripped away the interruptions and got you to your destination a lot sooner.

Now it all made sense why I had to go through the agony of a broken heart. I could never dedicate my life to training, hiking, and getting other people outdoors if I had to worry about a boyfriend.

I resolved to be single, and I focused on the trail.

3

BREW

AUGUST 2007—FEBRUARY 2008

Two weeks after swearing off relationships, I spent some time with my brother and his former college housemate. As much as I love my brother, I never thought that I would fall for one of his friends. But, after spending one afternoon with Brew, I knew that he was the best man I would ever meet. It was love at first hike.

Even so, a part of me still wanted to hold on to the "single and focused" plan. In fact, after Brew and I went on our first date together, a three-mile walk, I said good-bye, got in my car, and immediately started to vent.

"Really God? What about *our* plan?" I was both confused and unbelievably happy.

My fists were tensed, and adrenaline coursed through me. In a fit of excitement and frustration, I drummed on my steering wheel with sweaty palms.

Then I looked over and realized Brew was still standing in the parking lot, watching me. He smiled and waved. I turned beet red, slunk down in my seat, and drove off as quickly as possible.

Despite my friends' warning that Brew was a rebound boyfriend, and knowing that two weeks prior I had sworn off relationships, everything about being with Brew felt right. Typically, I was the queen of internalization, self-talk, and weighty dilemmas, but I had no doubts about my relationship with him.

Brew and I connected spiritually and emotionally, and we played together really well. In fact, we skipped the traditional dinner and movie ritual and instead spent our one-on-one time on "play dates." We got to know one another sweating on the tennis court, trash-talking under a basketball net, battling over board games, and conversing on the trail. It was a fun, active, and competitive courtship. Everything seemed to be perfect. We both loved sports, we loved the outdoors, and we both loved hiking. Well, Brew *thought* he loved hiking.

Brew was a recreational hiker. He liked to take his time, smell the roses, and venture out in relatively good weather. After a week of dating, Brew and I spent Labor Day climbing Mount Mitchell, the tallest mountain east of the Mississippi River. Of course, I picked the longest, most difficult route to the top. We made it to the summit and back down to the trailhead just as dusk turned into darkness, and when we reached the parking lot, I had a huge toothy grin on my face. However, Brew was groaning, limping, and cradling his groin to prevent further chafing.

"We did it!" I exclaimed.

Brew replied, "I have been praying that I would meet a girl who was outdoorsy, but I didn't mean *this* outdoorsy!"

Despite our different approaches to hiking, Brew always encouraged my trail pursuits. It never bothered him when I spent a day running and hiking on trails by myself or planned an overnight on my own. He was content to have a general idea of where I was going, when I would finish, and when he could see me again.

However, his enthusiasm wavered after John and Irene Bryant, an elderly couple from my hometown, were killed on a hike in the Pink Beds area of Pisgah National Forest west of Asheville. Brew became concerned for my safety and I couldn't blame him, even though I knew that statistically I was safer hiking down the trail than driving down the interstate. So, for the first time since I started backpacking, I began looking over my shoulder.

I felt scared and violated. I hated knowing that two people had been murdered on a trail where I had enjoyed outings as a child. Someone had damaged my emotional connection with a place that I associated with good friends, open meadows, and a rare and very beautiful pink water lily. I would never again be able to hike the trail, play in the meadows, or look at those lilies without thinking of the murders that took place there.

Even though the deaths of John and Irene Bryant happened in my backyard, they didn't hit home like the murder of Meredith Emerson. Meredith went missing on New Year's Day in 2008. She had gone hiking with her dog on Blood Mountain, Georgia, and when she didn't come home, the newspaper headlines throughout the southeast read, "Twenty-Four-Year-Old Female Hiker Missing Near A.T." Because I was twenty-four years old and frequently hiked on and near the Appalachian Trail, friends began calling me to make sure I was not the woman who had gone missing.

I initially felt connected to Meredith because of our age and gender, but as the details of her life were released, I was startled to realize how much we had in common. Our studies, hobbies, and faith paralleled one another. For the next five days, every morning I would go in to work and read the online headlines about Meredith's disappearance. The authorities concluded early on that she had been forcibly abducted. And as new details emerged each day, I would read the updates with tears streaming down my face. I had never experienced a news story that seemed so personal. I felt like Meredith was a close friend, and I didn't understand how this could happen to her. There was a sick emptiness in my stomach that said it could easily have been me.

The day that the authorities found Gary Michael Hilton and announced that he had in fact murdered Meredith, a deep ache consumed my core. I needed to cry and clear my head, and I needed to hurt. I went for a long, difficult hike. But even in the forest, something didn't feel right. The birds and the squirrels were quiet and still. It was as if all of creation were grieving.

To me, it seemed like Meredith's life was taken at the worst possible time. I knew the potential of a twenty-four year old; the potential of a new career and the opportunity to explore the world and see new places. The potential to fall in love, get engaged, and have your father walk you down the aisle—the hope that one day you would have children of your own. It was as if Gary Michael Hilton had robbed the world of a flower that was just about to bloom.

In the following days, as the news continued to unfold, it became clear that authorities had not simply happened upon Gary Michael Hilton. Meredith had left a path for them to follow. She had physically and mentally fought her captor at every turn. She used self-defense to fight him on Blood Mountain, which resulted in evidence that police used against him. She provided the wrong ATM pin number at several different locations to create an electronic trail. She had done everything right. She demonstrated a rare bravery and intelligence under those extreme circumstances.

Once Hilton was apprehended, he was charged with the murders of John and Irene Bryant near Asheville, and that of Cheryl Haines in a Florida national forest. He also became a suspect in several other missing person cases throughout the southeast. Meredith may not have been able to save herself, but she was responsible for saving the lives of many others and bringing some peace to the families of the victims.

I am grateful that the media decided to follow Meredith's story beyond her death, because it became clear that her legacy and influence had not ended. I know that it allowed me—and many others who felt like they knew Meredith—to heal.

I believed that because Meredith was a fighter and because she loved hiking and the wilderness, she would never have wanted her story to be something that kept other people from experiencing nature. Meredith reinforced my desire to get other people outside. She also reinforced my personal longing to explore the trails. So I decided that I would still try to set the women's speed record on the Appalachian Trail that summer, and I would do it in Meredith's honor.

To get ready for Appalachian Trail, I knew I needed to complete a substantial training hike, and I needed to practice hiking long days in hot weather. But in the months of January and February, that was all but impossible in North America. I had saved up money and vacation time, and I decided that at the end of January, I would travel to Australia and complete the six-hundred-mile Bibbulmun Track.

The problem with traveling halfway around the world to hike a trail without cell-phone service is that it made my boyfriend of five months extremely nervous. However, as an unmarried woman, I had to uphold certain standards in my relationship. And I refused to compromise or delay any adventures unless I was engaged.

In my previous relationship, Nightwalker had begged and pleaded for me not to go without him on a two-week hiking excursion to Peru. But he could not give me any date or idea of when he would be free to go, so I went on my own. Looking back, if I hadn't taken the initiative and traveled without him, I probably never would have gone to Cotahuasi Canyon or Machu Picchu, the sacred city of the Incas. And I would have regretted it.

So despite the fact that the past five months had seen several trail murders, and knowing that Brew would be worried sick about me while I was away, I disregarded the overwhelming feeling that I didn't want to be separated from my boyfriend for even a second, and I booked a four-week trip to Australia.

It turned out to be one of the smartest things I had ever done, because the week before I left, Brew gave me a ring.

He didn't want to be left out of my planning or my adventures ever again.

Hiking is, by definition, simply walking in a natural setting. But in reality, it is far more than that. It is a time of preparation and renewal. And in my opinion, the more fast-paced and over-stimulated the world becomes, the more important it will be to take a walk in the woods.

Traveling to Australia was heart wrenching because it put me 12,000 miles away from the person I loved most. But hiking the six-hundred-mile Bibbulmun Track was one of the best things I could have done for Brew, for myself, and for our impending marriage. Five months is a short time to date before getting engaged.

But instead of spending the first month of our engagement worrying about a wedding, I simply thought about marriage. I mourned the loss of my singleness and I contemplated the full meaning and commitment of matrimony.

Contemplation came easily, as the Bibbulmun Track was the most solitary trail I had ever hiked. Most Australians refuse to hike the footpath between December and February because of the one-hundred-degree heat. But after hiking through the southern California desert on the Pacific Crest Trail without any shade and very few water sources, the high temperatures on the Bibbulmun Track, which were often diffused by a forest canopy or ocean breeze, did not prove to be a problem for me.

During one stretch along my journey, I went three full days without seeing another person. A few years before, and certainly before I started hiking, that level of solitude would have made me really uncomfortable—or it simply would have driven me crazy. But now, I embraced the isolation and I embraced the crazy.

For three full days, I talked to animals instead of people.

The kangaroos were not very good conversationalists. They hopped off before I could even finish a sentence. In my first few days on the trail, I was constantly startled by the sound of them bounding through the underbrush. They were stronger, taller, and much faster than I expected—not nearly as quaint and cute as they'd been in the books I read as a child. But because I saw between fifteen and thirty a day, I quickly grew accustomed to them.

There were plenty of other critters. The emus reminded me of the ostriches that I had seen after climbing Kilimanjaro in Africa, but they were far more skittish. I usually spotted them near berry bushes, and as soon as they felt my presence, they panicked and sprinted off. The spiders in Australia were very large, but I actually preferred these giant arachnids to the smaller U.S. varieties because I could spot them from yards away, which kept me from hiking into so many webs. And then there were the lizards. They

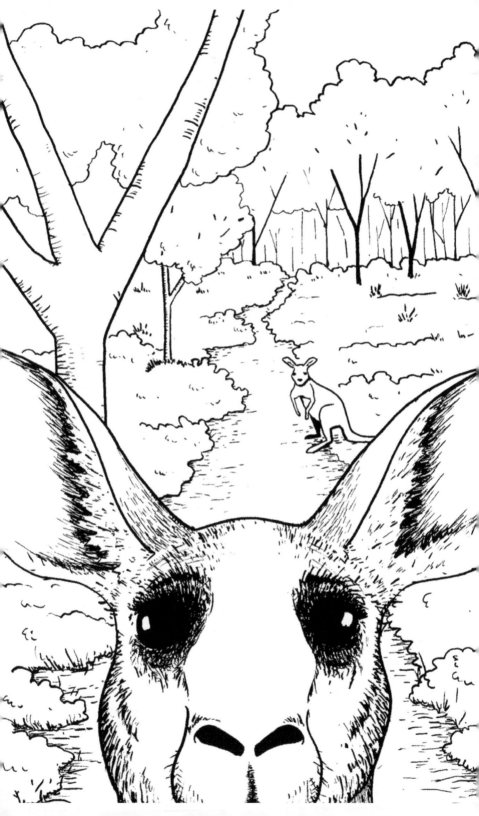

were so huge, colorful, and primitive that I was convinced I might also spot a dinosaur hiding in the forest.

Most of the human interaction I had occurred when I would reach a town and could call Brew on a payphone. He knew that I could call at any time, most likely during the middle of the night, so he didn't get very much sleep while I was on the Bibbulmun Track.

Hiking to hear Brew's voice encouraged me to hike longer days and higher miles. The reward for all my hard work was no longer reaching a warm shower or hot meal, but simply hearing my fiancé's voice. We both valued our time apart and recognized its significance in our relationship, but at the same time, we hated it.

One day toward the end of my hike when I reached the small town of Pemberton, I called Brew. It was late at night in the States, but I could tell his voice was weighed down with more than fatigue.

"I'm worried about this summer," he said.

"About the A.T.?" I asked hesitantly, knowing the answer.

In our brief planning session before my departure, we scheduled our wedding for June 8, right after Brew finished teaching and twelve days before I wanted to start the Appalachian Trail. I had told him on our first date that I was planning on a record attempt that summer, and I didn't want to give it up, especially now that I had dedicated it to Meredith. But looking down, I noticed the shiny new ring on my finger, and I realized I would have to try something that I wasn't very accustomed to—compromise.

Brew continued, "I just want to be able to see you as much as possible on the trail, and I can't imagine seeing you hurt or hungry or cold or wet, without being able to help you."

I took a deep breath. One thing Brew wanted assurance of before we got engaged was that I loved him more than hiking, and that I would always put him above the trail. In my mind—and my heart—there was no comparison, but he still needed to hear that.

"I want to do what is best for us," I said. "If that means that I don't get to hike the A.T. this summer, then I'll deal with it. But I've been dreaming about this trail record for months and working toward it. We are going to have our entire lives to be together and hike together, and I may not have the time or the ability to go after this record in the future. So I'd really like to do it now. Remember, you *are* robbing the cradle."

Brew's solemness eased, and he let out a laugh.

I liked to tease him that I was his trophy wife. I also liked to remind him of our five-year age difference and of the fact that he'd had his entire twenties to travel and explore. Marriage would certainly be our greatest adventure, but I still wanted to have some smaller exploits along the way.

"Well, what if we did a supported hike?" Brew asked.

"You mean you'd help me the whole way?"

I had never done a supported hike before. I had always traveled on my own with everything I needed on my back. In a supported hike, Brew would take our car and meet me at points where the trail crossed a road. I could limit my pack weight and have daily access to food, dry socks, and my husband. I loved the solitude and self-sufficiency of traditional backpacking, but I loved Brew more. It made sense that this would no longer be my hike, but our hike.

"I'm going to be following you and worrying about you anyway, so I might as well help you. What do you say? Want to try a supported record?"

And from half a world away I said, "I do."

· 4 ·

THE HONEYMOON

B rew and I were married on June 8, 2008, in a beautiful outdoor ceremony in the Blue Ridge Mountains near Charlottesville, Virginia. We spent almost two weeks honeymooning in Montpelier, Montreal, and Maine's Acadia National Park, and then on June 20, we began our supported thru-hike on the Appalachian Trail at Mount Katahdin, Maine. It was the greatest newlywed adventure that I can imagine, but it was also the most demanding.

The goal was to cover the Appalachian Trail's fourteen states and 2,180 miles in less than two months. My job was to wake up with the sun, hike all day, then go to bed when the sun went down. Brew's role was far more complicated.

I needed my new husband to locate obscure road crossings, hike in to find me, and always have the correct provisions in his pack or in the car. His role included setting up camp at night, preparing our food, running our errands, and encouraging me with positive feedback and humor whenever we were together.

At the end of the day Brew would sometimes hike in to meet me with our camping gear. Other times he would leave the last road crossing of the day with me and carry a pack with our supplies so that we could stop and set up camp. Ideally, if I could end the day at a road crossing, he would have our dinner ready, our tent set up, and our sleeping pads and bags unrolled by the time I arrived. It was up to him to make sure that I had everything I needed, all the time.

And I didn't realize how stressful the endeavor would be on Brew. He had never spent a night on the Appalachian Trail before the summer of 2008, and I had forgotten how difficult that transition could be. Brew had to grow accustomed to sleeping every night in a tent, waking up to black flies and mosquitoes buzzing in his face, and going several days without taking a shower. He also had to adjust to a diet of Clif bars and freeze-dried dinners. In other words, he had to learn to be very uncomfortable, very quickly.

But Brew's emotional burden was even greater than his physical discomfort. He had to learn simultaneously how to be a new husband *and* a one-man support team. On the trail, my success and safety depended entirely on Brew. If he couldn't find me, then I would not have any food or camping gear for the next section. My well-being was completely in his hands—and he knew it. And the fact that we started in the most logistically challenging and remote portion of trail didn't help his anxiety.

The northern terminus of the Appalachian Trail is in the middle of Maine, which is to say, the middle of nowhere. Katahdin, a large rocky monolith whose name means "Greatest Mountain," rises from the surrounding bogs and forests like an impenetrable fortress. It offers fulfillment to the thru-hikers who arrive at its base and hope to those who depart from its peak. The mountain is a great teacher, but its answers are always changing and are often bestowed in the form of new questions.

The day we began, I climbed the barren slopes of the Mighty Mountain with my new husband and then descended the arduous terrain on my own. After just a few hours, I exited the sanctuary of Baxter State Park. I paused at the park boundary and looked over my shoulder at the mountain behind me. I didn't know when I'd see it again, but I sensed that someday I would.

Ahead of me, Brew waited at the next road crossing. When I saw my husband standing at our car, I ran to meet him. He was my moving mountain, my migrating trail marker, a source of strength. Every time we parted, I would immediately look ahead and press forward to meet him again. Even on day one, it seemed that the motivation to set a record was less compelling than the incentive of hiking to Brew. At this point I was still thinking more about our wedding and our honeymoon than about the difficult task that lay ahead. I was too full of love to worry about the hardships of the next 2,000 miles.

I gathered more food and supplies at our car and kissed my husband good-bye before entering the Hundred-Mile Wilderness. The common misperception about the Hundred-Mile Wilderness is that there are not any roads for evacuation, entry, or support. But it only feels that way. The thick woods, low-lying marshes, large undisturbed lakes, and abundant moose make the wilderness seem remote and impassable. But there are roads. Granted, they are mostly unmarked private logging roads that you have to pay to access and pray to navigate, but there *are* roads.

Brew did a great job maneuvering through the maze of obstacles in the Hundred-Mile Wilderness and I was able to see him at least twice a day. After I hiked out of it and crossed the wide channel of the Kennebec River, access to the trail increased, and I could see Brew even more often.

When the burly climbs, copious river crossings, and swarming black flies of central Maine began to wear on my body and spirit, I could always count on Brew to sing me a song, tell me a joke, or give me a kiss that would get me through the next section.

There were multiple times when I was between road crossings, all alone, and my body felt like it couldn't take another step. In those moments, I would start to sing—poorly and out loud—the Diana Ross chorus, "Ain't no mountain high enough, ain't no valley low enough, ain't no river wide enough to keep me from getting to you." And my determination to overcome everything to get to my husband was renewed.

Brew felt the same way about finding me. Together we were a well-oiled machine, leap-frogging one another with perfect precision . . . until day six. That morning, I left early from our campsite near the still waters at Horns Pond Lean-to. Brew was still asleep in the tent, but I knew that in another hour, his alarm would sound and he would quickly pack up and hike down the mountain as well. I hiked four miles down a steep incline to where our car was parked at Maine Route 27. I changed clothes and loaded up on snacks for nine more miles of rugged terrain before I could see Brew and have access to our SUV again.

I made it to Caribou Valley Road in three hours, but when I arrived, Brew wasn't there. We had agreed to leave notes for each other on pieces of bright orange surveyor's tape in case one of us arrived early and had to press on. I looked around for one of those, but I could not find any on the nearby trees. The road was a rocky mess and had suffered multiple washouts from a nearby stream. It seemed like it would be difficult for an ATV to navigate, let alone a full-sized vehicle. I waited for Brew for over forty minutes. There were several times when I thought I heard our faithful Toyota Highlander traveling down the uneven road, and I was convinced that I could see a cloud of dust materializing through the trees, but the noise never grew louder and the car never appeared.

I had to make a decision. I either needed to start a twenty-four-mile stretch of very difficult terrain with a single granola bar in my pack, or I would have to waste more time waiting for Brew at a forest road that I was not convinced he could find or maneuver.

I heard a noise coming from inside the forest and looked up to see a thru-hiker exiting the trees. In spite of the difficulty of my own hike, I loved seeing the northbound thru-hikers in Maine. They were dirty, smelly, and hairy, and yet, at the same time, they were positively glowing. Most of them had been hiking now for three or four months and were within two weeks of their ultimate goal—Katahdin.

I smiled at the young man who had a bandana on his head and mud smeared across the inside of his ankles.

"Hey, there," he said. "I didn't expect to see a day hiker out here."

"Well, I am waiting for my husband. He was supposed to meet me here, but I'm worried he might be lost or might not be able to get our car down the road."

The thru-hiker looked around, his gaze lingering on the narrow, rocky, washed-out roadbed. He gave me a hopeless look.

"What are you going to do?" he asked.

"Well, I would keep going and try to reach Route 4, but I don't have enough food."

The thru-hiker grinned. He immediately took off his pack and began to dig inside, and after a few seconds, he pulled out an unopened pack of Chips Ahoy cookies. He said, "Here," and offered them to me.

"No, no, no. There's no way I could take food from a thru-hiker," I said.

"I can resupply in nine miles. You would be doing me a favor by lightening my load. Really, just think of it as trail magic."

Random acts of kindness that occur on the Appalachian Trail are part of what make the journey so special. And they often do more for your soul than your stomach. Generally thru-hikers with heavy backpacks fall on the receiving end of trail magic. But there I was, a supported hiker with a car full of gear and food somewhere in the vicinity, and I was receiving much-needed food from the least likely candidate. I could not believe this hiker's generosity or my good fortune. I accepted the cookies and thanked him.

I wrote a quick note to Brew on orange surveyor's tape, telling him I was okay and that he should hike in to meet me from the next road crossing. Then I stood up to leave the patch of sweet-smelling conifer trees where I had been sitting and started pacing down the trail, shoving cookies in my mouth and thanking God for the kind young man with the extra food.

For the rest of the day, I no longer worried about my well-being or safety; I only worried about Brew. Even though I didn't have a headlight, I knew if I kept my pace up, I could make it to the next road before dark. Brew, on the other hand, was potentially lost, having car trouble, and he was worried about the person he loved most being on an unforgiving stretch of trail with one granola bar and no flashlight.

In my head, I could see Brew cursing loudly as he drove down the back roads of western Maine, mad at himself for not being able to find me and worried sick that I was in trouble. Once I made it over the top of Saddleback Mountain, I began to run down the steep, rocky backside of the slope, hoping to reach my husband as quickly as possible.

A mile and a half before coming to the road, I saw Brew walking uphill toward me with a full pack on his back and two LED headlamps hanging around his neck. I could tell he had prepared to hike all night. When he spotted me running down the trail, he ran toward me too, jostling all of his gear. As we embraced, I could feel a warm, wet tear roll down our pressed cheeks, but I was uncertain whether the tear was his or mine.

We held each other for several minutes, then walked hand in hand to the road. Physically, it had been a long, hard day, but my body felt okay—aside from the fact that I could not imagine eating another chocolate chip cookie. It was my emotions that were wrecked. And Brew, who had been lost and worried for most of the day, was equally worn down.

That night we drove to a hotel in nearby Rangeley, where we got to shower, recover, and hold each other close in a clean, soft bed instead of sticking to each other inside our dirty sleeping bags.

I knew that there would be other places on the trail where we would cross wires or miss one another again, but now I also trusted that we would eventually be able to find one another, and I was confident that Brew would do whatever it took to reach me.

After overcoming the trauma of not being able to find me in the bowels of backcountry Maine, Brew joked that his error was actually a ploy that forced me to hike faster and farther. It was funny but completely untrue. Throughout the entire record attempt, Brew never pushed me. Every decision to rest, slow down, speed up, or increase my miles was my own.

Self-monitoring was tough. I had no clue what type of effort or exertion was required on a record attempt of over two thousand miles. I wanted to give my all, but I didn't know what my all was. I wanted to try and avoid overuse injuries, even though I was making the same motion and using the same muscles for ten to twelve hours a day. Like most hikers, trail conditions and the weather forecast factored into my daily mileage goals. The women's A.T. record stood at eighty-eight days. An unsupported hiker who carried all her gear set it in 1993. It was a far cry from the men's supported mark of forty-seven days. Women had not actively pursued a supported record—until now.

I was constantly taking stock of my health and wellness. On the trail, without the assistance of medical studies, on-call physicians, or WebMD, I resorted to listening to my body. I did not know what was "normal." I just knew that my goal was to hike over thirty-five miles every day.

When I left Maine, my body was not happy. I was covered in scrapes and bruises and my left ankle was red, swollen, and stiff. It had been irritated and in pain since the Hundred-Mile Wilderness. Over a week later, it still resembled a small ruby-red grapefruit. I didn't remember spraining it, but after turning and twisting the joint over uneven terrain for more than thirty miles every day, the cumulative effect felt worse than the sharp pain of any single misstep.

I decided that I would leave the trail and seek medical attention if the injury got worse. But because of my experience on the Long Trail and other long-distance paths, I also knew that I could hike through a lot of pain and even heal in the process. For a full week, my ankle didn't improve or become worse. Then, finally, when I made it to Pinkham Notch in New Hampshire, it started to feel better.

My body could not have picked a better point to mend itself. Pinkham Notch is a deep valley located between the high summits of Carter Dome and Mount Washington. And if there is any mountain of the Appalachian that makes you pray for good health and good weather, it is Mount Washington.

Mount Washington is a 6,288-foot peak located on top of a steep slope that resembles a rockslide. It is not the highest mountain on the trail in elevation, but for many hikers it presents the toughest climb. The path leading to the top leaves the protection of the forest—a boundary known as tree line—seven miles before the summit. From that point forward, the hike is a treacherous, hair-raising traverse over narrow ridges and loose rocks. It can be difficult to locate the trail on Mount Washington in good weather and impossible to find your way in inclement conditions.

In 2005, my hike up and down Mount Washington had been magical. I was traveling with my hiking companions Mooch and Nightwalker. The wind was strong, but the skies were clear and blue. The technical hiking on the mountain caused us to take our time, take pictures, and take solace in the fact that we were hiking the longest stretch of exposed terrain along the Appalachian Trail with good friends and without a storm in sight.

But this time, I found myself hiking up the same mountain alone, amid strong gusts of wind and dense fog. For five solid hours, I was terrified that I would get lost in the white blanket that covered every nook and cranny of the mountain. And if I did become lost, the steep precipices and late season snowfields on the mountain would leave me feeling like I might never be found. For ten miles I fought fear and uncertainty. My steps were short, my breathing was shallow, and I prayed constantly.

I didn't stop at the observatory on top of Mount Washington, nor did I duck out of the harsh conditions at the sheltered Lake-of-the-Clouds Hut. I was too worried that if I did stop hiking —even for a moment—I would lose the desire and courage to continue down the trail. It wasn't until I made it back into the protection of the forest that I collapsed in exhaustion.

Even through three layers of clothing, my heart still seemed to be beating out of my chest. I pulled some crackers, cheese, and dried fruit out of my pack and began to shove them into my mouth. I had spent the past eleven miles trapped in a tunnel of white fog and fear, and I had forgotten to eat.

I quickly took in calories, and I thought back to my encounter with Andrew Thompson on my first thru-hike. Andrew was on the trail in 2005, attempting to set the overall Appalachian Trail record. He eventually succeeded, and when I crossed paths with him on this rugged mountain, I knew why. Since we were above tree line between Mount Washington and Pinkham Notch, I was able to watch Andrew glide easily uphill toward me for fifteen minutes. I was struck by his presence even before I knew what he was doing. He was handsome and tall, with the strength of an ox and the grace of a ballet dancer, all while hiking over giant rocks. And as he approached, I could see his long, toned muscles glistening under a thin layer of sweat. But the physical attribute that stood out most on this Adonis was his smile.

Why in the world was he smiling? How was it possible for anyone to hike forty-six miles a day over unforgiving terrain and still smile?

Thinking about Andrew brought a small upward curl to my crumb-covered lips. I couldn't fathom the physical exertion of his record. I was hiking ten miles less per day than he had and it was still the most difficult challenge of my life. But there had been something in his smile that implied the challenge was worth it.

When I reached the road at Crawford Notch, I saw a very relieved expression on my husband's face. Before leaving the oasis of our car, Brew picked up a pack with our tent, two sleeping bags, two suppers, and lots of snacks, and together we continued hiking.

Even though the access roads in New Hampshire were paved, with far more amenities than the narrow dirt tracks in Maine, they never seem to intersect the trail at a good time. Usually by mid-afternoon, Brew would have to load an overnight pack and hike in with me so that my miles could stay consistent and so that I could maximize my hiking during daylight hours. These stretches quickly became my favorite part of the day.

The miles and the time flew by when I hiked with Brew. I recognized how special and unique this time together was, especially as newlyweds. Even though the terrain through the White Mountains offered some of the most challenging and perilous ascents and descents on the trail, I hardly noticed the steep grade when I hiked with Brew.

I was savoring the experience and my husband's companionship as we climbed up the wooden steps and metal handrails that dotted North Kinsman. Looking back, I said, "Think about it, Brew. We are away from our family, away from our friends. We have all this time to just be together. I mean *really* be together. We are learning how to communicate better and how to trust each other more fully. We are so fortunate to have this time together."

Brew looked up at me. Sweat was streaming off his forehead and soaking his gray t-shirt. The pack on his back, which had been built for me, looked crooked and top-heavy with our gear and food.

Half-jokingly, he asked, "Couldn't we have spent time away from our family and friends and developed our relationship more fully in Fiji?"

I was constantly reminded that while I was living out my dream, Brew was just along for the ride. And it was a long, hard, bumpy ride.

The trail remained constant in the sense that it was ever changing. Each day presented new obstacles, new logistics, and new miles to overcome.

Brew was experiencing the trail for the first time, but for me there was a part of the journey that felt familiar—even nostalgic and redemptive.

The first time I completed the Appalachian Trail, it had been a life-changing experience. Positive life-changing experiences are great in retrospect. But it hurts to be molded and made new, especially when you are as stubborn as I am.

In 2005, I was an inexperienced backpacker and I made every mistake possible on my journey from Georgia to Maine. Beyond having to overcome my own ineptitude, the trail conditions proved especially challenging for me.

The most horrific day of my 2005 thru-hike came at Sunrise Mountain, New Jersey, where I discovered the body of a young man who had committed suicide. In fact, there was a 0.2-mile piece of the Appalachian Trail that I still hadn't seen because after I called 911 and the authorities arrived, they rerouted me off the trail to provide a wide berth around a scene that had already imprinted itself in my mind in perfect detail.

Going back to the place where it happened was one of reasons I wanted to hike the trail again. I wanted to hike the entire trail, every last 0.2-mile section of it. But more than that, I wanted peace and I needed closure.

This time, when I reached New Jersey, Brew and I walked to the top of Sunrise Mountain together and sat down on a bench inside the pavilion where I had found the body. We held hands and looked out over the green plains that stretched toward the horizon. Brew and I both thanked God for the beauty of the surrounding area, then we remembered the young man who I had discovered three years earlier and we prayed for his family and friends.

After praying, Brew wrapped his arm around my shoulder. I nuzzled my head into the crook of his arm. We were silent for a minute as we listened to the soft breeze blowing across the ridge. I felt courageous coming back to that mountain, and surprisingly, I also felt peaceful and safe.

"Are you okay?" asked Brew.

I nodded slowly.

"What are you thinking about?"

"Well, I am thinking about the suicide and Gary Michael Hilton—and about Meredith. I am reminded that things can end, and that life can end, very quickly. It makes me want to keep going."

"Well then you better go," whispered Brew.

I stood up and took several confident steps away from the pavilion before looking back over my shoulder to see Brew still sitting there, watching me walk away. His eyes were filled with love.

I paused to take in all the details of the scene: the light-blue sky, the purple flowers peeking through the rocky terrain, my husband's green shirt and scruffy beard. Making a new memory on top of that mountain eased the fear and pain that the summit once represented. When I turned to continue hiking, my breaths felt full and deep, and my footsteps felt light. I was reminded that my ability to succeed on the trail wasn't just about reducing the physical weight that I carried; it was about reducing the emotional weight as well.

In the mid-Atlantic states, Brew combined his support role with a historic driving tour of Appalachia. He visited West Point near Bear Mountain, New York, and he saw Gettysburg when I hiked through the Cumberland Valley in Southern Pennsylvania. Often, I would string together a slew of short sections without support so that Brew could go exploring. Most of the time, he returned from his excursions and waited for me at the designated trailhead for thirty minutes to an hour. But there were a few times when *I* had to wait for *him*.

At one road crossing in Pennsylvania, I had to wait twenty minutes. And I was famished. I had just hiked an eighteen-mile stretch that easily could have been split into three different sections. But Brew had wanted to travel to Pottsville to tour the famous Yuengling Brewery, which, as Brew pointed out, was still a historical site since it is the oldest brewery in America. And that was all well and good, but now he was late.

Not only was I hungry, but I was also parched. The "seasonal springs" located on the previous eight-mile stretch were all out of season. Usually, when I was dehydrated, I refused to cry because I knew it would result in losing more water. But my overwhelming need to eat and drink combined with the knowledge that Brew was delayed because he was at a tasting room caused my tears to pour like a barroom tap.

When Brew finally arrived, my face was beet red. Paths of salt traced their way down my dusty cheeks like dried riverbeds. Receiving food, water, and an apology made me feel better momentarily, but overall—regardless of Brew's words or actions—I was struggling.

Pennsylvania is a hard state to hike through. You feel like you should be elated because you have finished half the trail, over 1,000 miles. But in the back of your mind, you know that the last 1,000 miles was the hardest challenge you have ever had to overcome, and now you are tired, and even more homesick and you still have another 1,000 miles to go. The glass feels half-empty in Pennsylvania.

Beyond the emotional and mental difficulty of Pennsylvania, the Appalachian Trail in this mid-Atlantic state comprises mostly of rocks. It is as if all the other states took all their rocks and dumped them here. Every step in Pennsylvania is a transfer of weight from one sharp, jagged rock to another. Since leaving New York, the pain in my feet and the large callus on my left big toe increased every day. Even my neck started to ache from always looking down at the virtual quarry beneath my feet.

After traversing nearly two hundred miles of the Appalachian Trail in Pennsylvania, I felt depleted. The rocks on the trail in the one-hundred-degree heat felt like charcoal on a grill, and I was the slow-cooking main course.

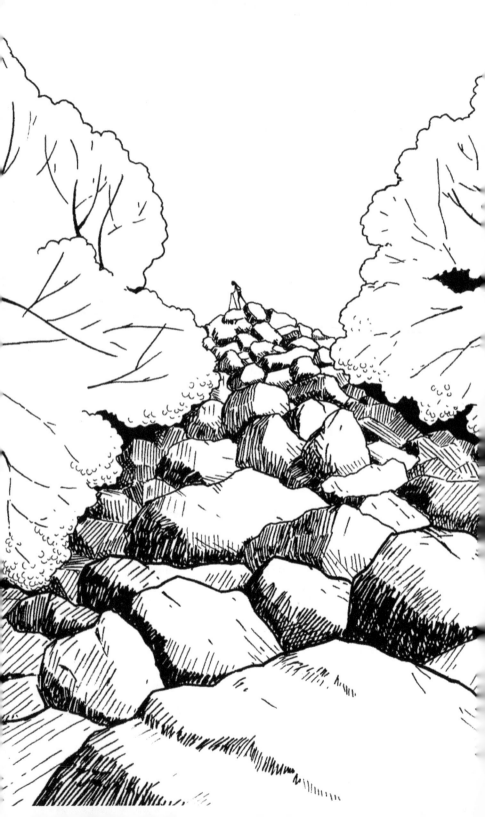

Brew had been late to a road crossing earlier in the day because he had been sipping beer at Yuengling. This time it was due to the tangled, unmarked roads, but it didn't matter. The fact that he missed me twice in one day accelerated my meltdown.

When he did finally show up, I was crying (again) and tossing small rocks into the woods. Rather than acknowledging him, I threw the small stone in my right hand toward a large rock that sat on the trail. Instead of hitting the intended target, the rock ricocheted off a nearby tree and hit me in the shin. I HATED rocks!

Then I turned toward my husband and, without giving Brew a chance to explain, I immediately expressed my displeasure—which sounded especially irrational since I hadn't had any food or water yet.

"Where were you?" I squawked. "I haven't had a snack in over six miles and my throat is so dry it hurts to breathe. Why weren't you here when I got here?!"

Brew stared at me for an eternity before opening his mouth. He's not one to raise his voice, and sometimes that makes his responses even louder. "Ever since the last road crossing, I have been driving down piss-poor, unmarked dirt roads trying to find you. And in case you were wondering, it wasn't much fun. *This* isn't much fun."

Then, after making sure I had gotten what I needed out of the car, Brew drove off without saying another word.

Things weren't much better between the two of us in Duncannon. We walked without speaking down the asphalt road that guides the Appalachian Trail through the small town. When we reached the car at the end of town where the path returns to the confines of the forest, I silently began to refill my water bottle and select my snacks for the next section. The stubbornness that allows me to hike all day every day without stopping is the exact same quality that forces my husband to initiate all of our reconciliations.

"I don't think you know how hard this is on me," he said.

Without looking up, I immediately replied, "I don't think you realize how hard this is on *me*!"

I could tell I had hurt Brew again, but that didn't stop me. He expected disagreements to be a discussion; I preferred a monologue.

"I just need more. I need to know you are giving this one hundred percent. This is the hardest thing I have ever done in my entire life, and when you are late to the road crossing or can't find my gear because the car is a mess—it makes a difference. It costs me time, and it stresses me out."

"I'm giving you everything I have."

I looked up at Brew. He had tears lining his eyelids. The sincerity and pain on his face transformed my anger into guilt.

Suddenly, I felt horrible.

"I'm, um, I am . . . I'm sorry," I sputtered. I took a minute to regroup my emotions and then I reached for his hand. "I know this is hard for you. I know you are doing your best."

Brew gave me a familiar look. He didn't like my apologies. He never thought that I said "I'm sorry" with the right tone. Coming from a background where you were lucky to get any sort of apology, I didn't understand what he was talking about.

"You better keep hiking," he said, his voice sounding wounded but stern. "You still have eight more miles, and if you don't leave now, the sun will go down while you are on the rocks."

I turned and started hiking uphill, out of Duncannon. And as I did, I realized that I didn't want the sun to set while I was on the rocks in Pennsylvania *or* on the rocks with my husband. I hiked as quickly as I could to the next road crossing, where I could give Brew a better apology.

While my feet sped down the trail, I thought back to some of the worst arguments we'd had before we got married. I was starting to notice a theme. There had been only a few of them, and all but one had happened on training runs of over thirteen miles. Most of our arguments weren't even real disagreements, they were outbursts caused by fatigue, low blood sugar, and a lack of fluids. But at this moment, the cause wasn't nearly as important as the resolution.

Four miles into an eight-mile stretch, I saw Brew hiking toward me. He had found a closer road and then hiked north. I started running over the scattered rocks.

"Don't run!" he called. He didn't want me to fall and get hurt, but he couldn't stop me from sprinting toward him. Within twenty seconds, I was in his arms, apologizing over and over again. I hoped that one of them would sound right. I would have done anything to show Brew that I was sorry. I would have quit right there if he had asked.

Brew tightened his grip on me. "I'm sorry too," he said. "I feel like I'm giving you everything out here. But if you need more, I will find a way to give you more."

From that point on, I never again questioned Brew's level of commitment.

Up until the Smokies, the few occasions when we had received additional help had been a luxury. But at Davenport Gap, it became a necessity. It was mid-August and I still had two-hundred forty-miles left to hike, but Brew had to go home and go back to work as a teacher.

He had been my physical and emotional support the entire trip, and I was heartbroken that he had to leave. We had been on the trail together for over fifty days, and now, with less than a week left, I couldn't imagine finishing the trail without him. We were both a wreck.

When I came out to Waterville School Road, our last road crossing together, I discovered that he had lost the keys to the car, and I couldn't get any provisions. Instead of being upset with Brew for being chronically disorganized—or for the fact that I would not be able to eat or drink—I simply leaned on my husband as he peered inside the windows to see if he could spot the keys. I didn't need food or water nearly as much as I needed my husband.

Brew convinced me to keep hiking another two and a half miles to Davenport Gap. He promised to find the keys and meet me there to say a final good-bye. When I arrived at the northern entrance to Smoky Mountain National Park, he was sitting in the car with the doors open, giving final instructions to his replacements.

Although Brew was leaving, I was not going to load up my backpack and complete the remainder of the trail on my own. My husband was sitting near the trail, instructing three sixty-year-old men on how best to provide support while he was away.

The fourth-quarter subs were a motley crew. Two of them were short and round, one with a permanent tan and silver hair, the other with a sideways ball cap and a white Santa Claus beard. The third member was tall, fit, and clean shaven and had a buzz cut. When they saw me coming down the trail, they all started to cheer.

I grinned. I don't think that we could have put together a more diverse team of men; I know for certain that we could not have found another trio of sixty-year-olds who I loved more.

The tall, svelte man who looked like a military officer was our friend David Horton. I had met him when he was sprinting up the muddy tread of a Virginia mountain named "The Priest" during a rainy morning on my initial A.T. hike in 2005.

Horton had set the overall Appalachian Trail record in 1991 by hiking the trail in fifty-two days. The summer after we met, he also set the record on the Pacific Crest Trail. Horton had also introduced me to ultra–trail running by inviting me to several of his races in Virginia. That's where I discovered that trail runners were a lot like thru-hikers. They loved the trail and a good challenge; they just usually had less time to be outdoors.

The man standing next to Horton with the light beard and crooked hat was none other than Warren Doyle. He had helped me prepare for my first A.T. hike, and we had crossed paths on the Pacific Crest Trail. He had also mentored me before my Long Trail record, and now he was here to assist me once again. He didn't wear Horton's smile of excitement, but instead looked thoughtful, almost stoic. Knowing him, I could just see the numbers floating around in his head. He was always calculating miles. It was one of the things he did best.

Warren had set the first endurance record on the trail in the 1970s by hiking the full distance in sixty-six days with limited support. Since then, he had hiked the entire A.T. more than fourteen times. For the next five days, he would be our logistics captain and back-roads navigator.

The final addition was my father. He didn't have the trail knowledge or experience that Horton and Warren had, but he would provide the intangibles and the emotional support that I needed. My dad was my first and biggest fan. He had encouraged me on my initial thru-hike of the Appalachian Trail and had driven up to Maine to meet me when I finished. And when I hiked the Pacific Crest Trail, he had flown out to Oregon to visit and feed me for three days. That time with him—along with the extra calories—provided the strength that I needed to reach Canada.

No matter what I did, and no matter where I traveled, I knew that my father was always in my corner.

The next four days, my mileages were higher than they had been the entire summer. I was invigorated by the new crew members.

Their constant encouragement and enthusiasm left me feeling far more energetic than I should have after hiking 2,000 miles. Plus, I knew that the sooner I finished the trail, the sooner I could reconnect with Brew.

Horton spent a lot of time on the path with me. Horton loves to run. Unfortunately for him, though, I spent most of my time hiking. For the most part, he tolerated it and stayed with me, but he also encouraged me to run—or at least jog—the downhill and flat sections.

"Let's run here. . . . This is a good place to run. . . . Don't you want to run?" He reminded me of a caged greyhound.

"Horton, I'm a hiker, not a runner."

"You are *too* a runner. You come to my races and you run and you finish with the top ten or fifteen women."

"Yeah, but I *think* like a hiker. Even at your races, I treat aid stations like trail magic, and I pass people who are running uphill just by hiking hard. I don't dream about running trail races; I dream about hiking long-distance trails."

"I still don't think you are a hiker. Hikers are lazy. Hikers always lose a lot of weight on the trail, but then after their thru-hikes, they stop exercising and they get fat. Look at Warren."

Horton was never one to watch his tongue or worry about what he said. This quality made him both offensive and endearing.

"Well, I like to move through the woods. I don't care how I do it. Maybe just think of me as a mover."

We kept moving until I arrived at the next road crossing. Warren was already waiting for me with a guidebook, atlas, and legal notepad. The Trail Yoda, as Brew liked to call him, encouraged me to sit down to eat and drink. And as I refueled, he described the next section of trail.

The visual aids spread before us were for me, not him. Warren never looked at his maps or notes when talking about the trail. He didn't have to. He had a photographic memory of the Appalachian Trail. He knew every climb, every switchback, and every spring. I trusted Warren more than I trusted a guidebook, and I usually based my water, food, and gear choices solely on his descriptions.

He stressed that the decision of how far to hike each day was my own, and that he was there only to provide me with options. Toward the end of each day, he would give me three or four choices for when to stop and where to camp. However, unlike Brew, I knew that Warren, Horton, and even my dad shared specific hopes and expectations for where I would stop. In other words, they pushed me. And I liked it.

The excitement of my three helpers never permitted me to stop early. My dad was especially proud of my success and eager to help me reach my final goal. And the constant stream of compliments and praise from Warren and Horton increased my father's nervous energy. Often he would turn on the car and start driving off to find the next road, sometimes before I even had a chance to restock my provisions.

I relished the brief interactions at the road crossings, not between the crew and me, but between the three men. They were so dissimilar. Their antics conjured up old black-and-white images of the Three Stooges, except my lovable modern-day men were running around and bumping into one another because they were trying to locate a lost map, find snack food, or decide which water bottle smelled less like fermented Gatorade. They communicated with each other incessantly and without awaiting a reply.

Although it wasn't always graceful, the interactions between them were surprisingly harmonious. And their antics got the job done.

Over the last four full days of my hike, I completed three forty-seven-mile stretches and capped them off with a sixty-five mile stretch into Neels Gap. I never thought I could complete

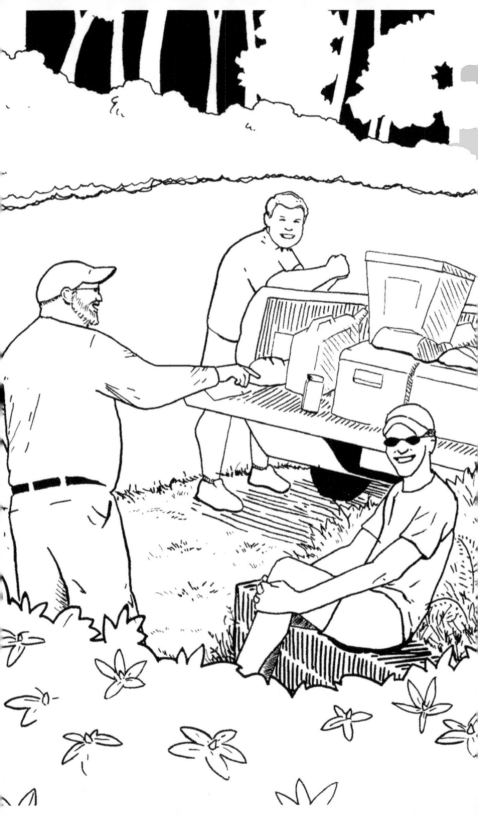

sixty-five miles in one day when I started this endeavor. But somewhere along the journey I learned that much of what I thought was impossible was simply very, very difficult.

There is a historic and well-known outfitter at Neels Gap known as Mountain Crossings, and when I reached the store just after dark on my last full day of hiking, the three men were beside themselves. Horton, despite having hiked over twenty-five miles with me that day, continued to pace around the parking lot.

"Thirty more miles, thirty more miles and you'll be on Springer Mountain. You're doing it, girl! You don't realize how special this is. You're doing it!"

Warren had his head bowed and was swaying gently back and forth almost as if he were in a trail-induced trance.

"*Sixty-five miles.* A sixty-five-mile day. Unbelievable."

My dad's beaming white smile was illuminated every five seconds by the flash of his camera.

Despite their theatrics, I barely noticed them. The only person I was focused on was Brew. He was back.

It was Friday night and Brew had driven from school to Georgia that afternoon to meet us. His presence made me feel complete. It wouldn't have been right to finish this hike without him.

The first and last day of a trail record are the easiest. My body ached and I was exhausted, but with less than thirty miles left to hike, I traveled the path effortlessly. In the miles leading up to Springer Mountain, I envisioned my friends and family waiting there in the parking lot.

In addition to my dad, Horton, and Warren, I knew that Brew's parents would be there as well. I tried not to think about the fact that my own mother would not be at Springer Mountain. Still, after almost five years, she still refused to come out to the trail because she was worried about my safety. I was hoping that she would get over her anxiety and support me this time, but I had gotten my stubbornness from my mother, so I knew not to expect her.

However, Maureen, my mom's closest friend, did make the trip to Springer Mountain. She often translated my mother's words and actions to me in a way that I could understand. That afternoon, Maureen did not try to explain my mother's absence; she simply offered her presence as a substitute.

From the parking area, it is only a one-mile hike to reach the top of Springer Mountain and the southern terminus of the Appalachian Trail. I wanted to share that journey with the people who had come to support me, but because of that, my last mile was one of my slowest all summer. It took us over forty minutes. At first, it was endearing how my father-in-law wanted to stop every twenty steps to look into the forest and examine a leaf, but halfway to the top, I decided I should have scheduled the group hike for our *return* to the parking area. I had been on the trail for fifty-seven days, hiking and running thirty-eight miles each day, and in that moment, all I wanted to do was reach the summit and finish the journey.

When we finally exited the forest, Brew and I walked hand in hand to touch the A.T. plaque on the gray boulder that crowned the mountain. It was one of the best feelings of my entire life. I was surrounded by friends and family, I had just completed my second thru-hike of the Appalachian Trail, and Brew and I had set the women's record on the trail.

After giving out hugs and taking pictures, we laid down on the sun-baked granite and took a twenty-minute nap. It wasn't your typical celebration, but for us it was the perfect finale to a wonderful adventure. And while there was no doubt that I was utterly exhausted, there was one little problem.

On our hike down to the Springer Mountain parking area, I kept thinking about how I could have kept going.

· **5** ·

THE DECISION

AUGUST 2009—JUNE 2011

When we set the women's record, Brew had several standard phrases that he would repeat along the trail, including, "It's a nice day to take a walk," "All you have to do is hike home," and my personal favorite, "Hike it out."

"Hike it out" meant that this was my one chance to do something great. This was the only time I would be able to attempt a record on the Appalachian Trail. It would also be the only time in our marriage when I would do what I wanted every day and Brew would follow me around, run our errands, and do my chores.

Looking back, I don't know if my husband would ever have agreed to such a difficult, thankless task if I hadn't planned the adventure directly after we got engaged. He signed on the dotted line at the height of infatuation. Because of that, there were several times during the summer when his devotion diminished and he seemed like he was having buyer's remorse.

However, Brew faithfully upheld his commitment, and when I thanked him and praised him and told him that as payback I would watch one hundred college football games with him on TV, bring him beer at any point, and rub his shoulders during half-time, he looked at me with a serious stare and then shook his head, saying, "No. Absolutely not. We are not quantifying this. I am holding this over you for *the rest of your life.*"

I truly believed that it was my last record—but not our last trail. I still wanted hiking to be a part of my life, and of our life together. As for my husband, he had sworn off supported hikes, but when it came to hiking side by side, Brew was ready to become a thru-hiker. His sampling of the Appalachian Trail made him want to travel a path from start to finish on his own two feet. So the following summer we headed west and completed the five-hundred-mile Colorado Trail together.

It was great—most of the time.

Brew had to go through the uncomfortable learning curve of his first thru-hike. The difficulty of carrying a heavy pack and the discomfort that resulted from hiking five days without taking a shower had become second nature to me. But Brew struggled with the pain in his shoulders, the blisters on his feet, and his sweaty dirty body parts sticking together inside a sleeping bag at night. It was hard for him. It was hard for most people. But unlike most people, Brew was fortunate because he had me there to tell him what to do.

That might have been our biggest challenge on the Colorado Trail. Not only had I forgotten how difficult it was to thru-hike without prior experience, but I also didn't remember how one of the most rewarding aspects of backpacking was learning how to become self-sufficient and make decisions on your own. We may have been walking side by side, but for the first week or two, it was still my hike.

I was deciding how many miles we would hike each day, and I was picking the exact spot where we would set up our tent at night. I chose all of our food at the resupply points and decided how many provisions we needed in order to reach the next town. I had determined our course of action on the Appalachian Trail and we had been successful. Trying to make decisions together on the Colorado Trail took a lot of communication and usually required a long explanation on my end. It was frustrating. What had become instinctual for me was still a thought-process for Brew. Things were just simpler when I called the shots.

Unlike me, Brew is a very good communicator, especially on the trail. And in Colorado, his discourse was dominated by the topic of discomfort.

"I have had wet feet for three days, and our tent is still soaked," Brew sulked. "Can't we take some extra time to dry everything out?"

"Why?" I countered. "Everything will just get wet again this afternoon when it rains."

"But what if it doesn't rain today?"

"It's rained every afternoon since we got out here—at least every afternoon that it hasn't hailed!"

"Yes, but you don't know that it will rain today. You don't know *everything!*"

I was silent. His comment had just slipped out, but it still hurt. And his honesty finally made me realize what a control freak I was being.

I'd learned how to thru-hike by making decisions and by making mistakes. Brew deserved that same opportunity. I needed to stop being the one who chose how many miles we hiked and where we camped. I needed to let Brew be the one to decide what food we would buy at our next resupply stop. That afternoon, we even stopped to dry out our tent and shoes . . . thirty minutes before the rain started to fall. Finally, we were headed in the right direction. But even after I gave Brew more ownership, he still kept talking.

One morning we were climbing up a grassy mountain slope. The birds were chirping and flitting in and out of the tall grass like rocks skipping over a still pond. I wanted to be present. I wanted to be in the moment and take it all in. But that was difficult when Brew was behind me, talking about his chronic chafing problems.

My frustration heightened along with our ascent. Finally, after thirty minutes of listening to the same complaints and potential cures that I had heard many times before, I looked back and said, "Brew, I love being with you, but you know we don't have to talk *all* the time, right?!"

"I'm not talking *all* the time," he said.

"Well, you're talking *a lot* of the time."

"I thought that was what you wanted." He paused (but just briefly). "You always talk about how much fun you had walking with Nightwalker and Mooch on your first A.T. hike. It seemed like your hike got a lot better when you started hiking and talking with them."

"Well, it did, but we still didn't talk *all* the time. We didn't even hike together most of the time."

"You didn't?"

"No, usually we all went at our own pace and then we met up to eat and camp together."

"Oh."

The way he responded, I suddenly realized that my husband hadn't been talking incessantly for his enjoyment; he had been doing it because he thought it was what *I* wanted.

After that, Brew was silent for a few minutes. And the next time he opened his mouth, he said, "Well, I'm not going to talk as much. But maybe I'll start singing more."

For the last two weeks of our hike, we continued hiking together most of the time, but we were quiet more. We both spoke up when we had something to say, and three or four times a day, Brew would sing out loud. He wasn't doing it to fill the silence; he was doing it because *he* enjoyed it. And I liked it, too.

I don't know of any situation where spouses, partners, or significant others spend more time together than on a thru-hike. Even if a married couple is working together, they will still spend time on their own. But hiking a trail with someone is like being tethered to him. You are dependent on one another for shared food and gear. You travel together during the day, and sleep in a small, enclosed tent at night. There is no personal space.

Completing the Colorado Trail was an invaluable experience for the two of us as individuals and as a couple. Brew had learned how to thru-hike, and I had learned how to thru-hike with someone else. And once again, the trail had strengthened our marriage. We had spent more quality time alone together, away from friends and family. Even if it hadn't been in Fiji.

When Brew and I finished our five hundred miles together, we were literally finishing each other's sentences. Before that trip, I didn't know that I still had so much to learn about my husband. And even though we felt completely in-sync, there was still one thing that I hadn't told him by the time we reached Denver.

As soon as we were off the Colorado Trail, Brew started making plans for the following year. I couldn't wait to spend another summer hiking with my husband, and this time, he was picking the trails, doing all the planning, and making all the decisions.

The problem was, he was picking trails in Europe, and my heart wanted to go back to the A.T.

Four months after our successful women's record, I had gone for a hike with Warren and he had asked me if I would ever consider trying for another trail record. I scoffed at him. I was done with records.

But then, a few months later, going on a long run by myself, I kept thinking of places on the trail where I could have saved time, where I could have hiked a longer day, or where we could have eliminated a mistake. I knew for a fact that I could do the A.T. better, more efficiently, and probably for a faster time. But in spite of that, I wasn't sure that I wanted to go back. Records were hard; they were trying on my body, on my emotions, and especially on my husband.

I was hoping the thought of returning to the A.T. for another record would go away. I thought it would disappear on the Colorado Trail, especially once Brew evolved into a decisive musical hiking partner, but the longing grew stronger and the questions in my head grew louder.

Now, my husband was planning our biggest, best summer of hikes ever—stops in Geneva and London with hikes in the Alps, the Scottish Highlands, and along the coast of Wales—and all I could think about was doing the A.T., and doing it in less than fifty-seven days. My soul was screaming and my mind was telling it to be silent.

When I was quite sure I could not quiet these nagging thoughts on my own, I went to the one person who I knew would put them to bed.

I was sure that if I brought up the idea of doing another record, Brew would squelch it immediately. And once he did, that would be the end of that.

So on a late-summer evening, as we walked hand in hand, I carefully broached the subject.

"Brew, I have a question."

"Yes . . . ?"

He could tell by the sound of my voice that this was not just any question.

"Do you think if I went back to the A.T. that I could do it better?"

"What do you mean by better?" he asked as he tilted his head toward me.

His probing stare left me wishing I could swallow the words that had just left my mouth. But once I had started, I had to keep going.

"Well, do you think I could do it faster?"

"Yes," Brew replied hesitantly. "I do."

I continued.

"Do you think I could do it in less than fifty-five days?"

"Probably."

"What about less than fifty days?"

"Maybe."

"What about forty-seven?"

Brew stopped walking and turned in my direction.

He finally realized the full scope of what I was asking, and I fully expected him to shoot it down. But instead, he said, "If everything fell into place, and you didn't get hurt, yeah, I think we could set the record."

We? That wasn't the response I was expecting; and I interpreted it as a divine miracle. But it also proved to be a curse. Now that the door of possibility cracked open to reveal a glimmer of light, the thought of going back to the trail consumed me.

After that discussion, I thought about the record every single day. I didn't mean to, and I didn't talk about it, but when things were silent and I started to daydream, my thoughts would always drift toward the trail. But it wasn't quite time to make a final decision. Not yet.

Instead, I agreed with Brew that we should enjoy another summer hiking side by side in Europe. Then, after more time and more miles had passed, we would revisit the A.T. discussion.

When Brew and I went to Europe, we began our hiking extravaganza on a long-distance trail in Corsica called the GR20. It was one of the most beautiful and difficult routes I had ever been on. I loved being on a trail again and I embraced the degree of difficulty, but Brew was not expecting the strenuous climbs.

Even worse, somewhere amid his planning, there was a discrepancy in the mileage, and after our second day of hiking we found that the GR20 was actually longer than we had anticipated. That meant we had to average close to twenty miles a day to finish on time. And that was not Brew's style of backpacking.

Midway through the trip, when we arrived at a rural campground that marked our one resupply stop, we were dismayed to discover a sparse pantry with only a few boxes of crackers, some cookies, and a stick of cured salami. We bought almost all the provisions they had, but I was still worried that it wouldn't be enough to keep us fed. Even if there had been more food, we would have been at a loss because we were out of euros, the store did not accept credit cards, and there wasn't an ATM in the town.

After our resupply, I visited the facilities and savored the only shower stall that we would encounter during our week-long trek. The narrow closet where I bathed was covered in mold and built for petite Europeans. My six-foot frame banged against the walls whenever I reached for shampoo or bent to pick up the soap. But I didn't care. It was still a shower.

When I was finished, so was the warm water. Without meaning to, I had left Brew nothing but an icy stream. I felt horrible, but there wasn't anything I could do to make it better. Instead, I continued to do chores like rinse out our clothes at a nearby water pump. After wringing out our shirts, shorts, and socks, I hung them on a fence and walked back to our tent. I could hear sniffling coming from inside the thin Silnylon walls.

I crawled into the shelter and started rubbing Brew's back. I knew what was wrong—"everything," according to my husband—but I asked anyway.

"Honey, what is it?"

"This is not how I thought it would be. My shower was freezing because you took all the warm water. I'm uncomfortable, our clothes are still dirty and now they're wet, my legs and crotch are chafing so badly that I can hardly walk, and I screwed up planning this hike."

"It'll be okay. Things will get better. We'll still be able to finish."

"You don't understand."

"What don't I understand?"

"This is still your thing. Not mine. I like the idea of backpacking, but I don't like doing it all day, every day. I want the views without so much hard work. I want the memories without feeling dirty and tired all the time. I want hot food and time to read books and take naps." Then Brew paused to wipe away the gleaming river of snot that was running through his beard. He looked up at me, and I could see the tears welling up in his eyes again. He put his hands over his face and declared, "I'm a *Romantic!*"

I tried as hard as possible not to let him see the tiny smile that was creeping across my face. It was true, Brew wanted things to be perfect, less painful. He was an idealist. But he was also becoming a pretty good backpacker, and that meant—despite the occasional meltdown—he was getting more comfortable being, well, uncomfortable.

"Honey, if I had all your issues right now, I would be crying too. You are a Romantic, but you are a *tough* Romantic."

Unfortunately, my words did not provide any immediate consolation to Brew's tender heart . . . or his tender crotch. It wasn't until the next day, after he'd had a good night's sleep, and after the sun had dried out our clothes and warmed our bodies, that we could joke about his romantic side.

Together, we made it through the GR20 in Corsica—arguably the toughest trail in Europe—in only seven days. To celebrate our finish we found an ATM, then a pub with cold beer, warm food, and World Cup soccer on TV. Despite all the modern amenities in front of us, all Brew could talk about was how amazing the trail had been. At the end of each hike that he completed, my husband became a little less Henry David Thoreau and a little more Daniel Boone.

After Corsica, we traveled to the Alps to hike the Tour du Mont Blanc. It became very clear to me on this one-hundred-mile circuit why people burst into spontaneous song in *The Sound of Music*. The Alps were perfect. The temperature was ideal, the views were amazing, there weren't any bugs, and every day we passed a small farm where we could pick up fresh cheese, cured meats, or local wine. It was the perfect place for a romantic hike—and a romantic hiker.

I cannot say the same for Wales. When we traveled to the southwest corner of the United Kingdom to hike the Pembrokeshire Coastal Path, we arrived during a medium downpour and then spent the next two and a half days hiking through a torrential storm. I have never been so wet in my entire life.

After the first day of slogging through inches of standing water, Brew made a decision.

"Listen, if this keeps up, I am not going to finish this trail. You can do whatever you want. I am fine if you want to keep walking, and I can just meet you every few days or at the end or whatever. But if I have to go through another day of this, I'm done."

I knew my husband was sincere, but I also believed the rain would stop. I didn't think it was possible for that much water to continue falling from the sky.

Twenty-four hours later, we were still walking through a wall of rain. Brew and I hadn't said much all day. I was miserable, and I assumed I would be on my own after that evening. Our guidebook, which was soaking wet, with pages glued together by the rain and ink running everywhere, suggested that toward the end of the day we would come to a town. We both assumed that when we arrived there would be a pub, or a bed and breakfast, or even a public restroom where we could briefly escape from the rain.

As night fell, we reached the town to discover three small houses and a bus stop. Desperate, we knocked on the door of one of the houses. A man with white hair, red cheeks, and fine wrinkles on his face opened the door. His stare suggested that he was both taken aback and also empathetic to our haggard appearance.

Without wasting time, Brew immediately said, "We're sorry to bother you, but is there a hostel or pub anywhere in the area where we can get out of the rain."

The man shook his head no, then after a pensive moment, he smiled and offered in his thick Welsh accent, "You are welcome to stay in my barn if you want."

We immediately accepted. The man then put on his raincoat and, with his border collie by his side, led us through a nearby field to his barn. The building was made of rocks and clay and had a packed dirt floor, but it also had four sides and was divided into rooms so we could sleep separate from the sheep and cows. Finally, we were out of the wind and rain.

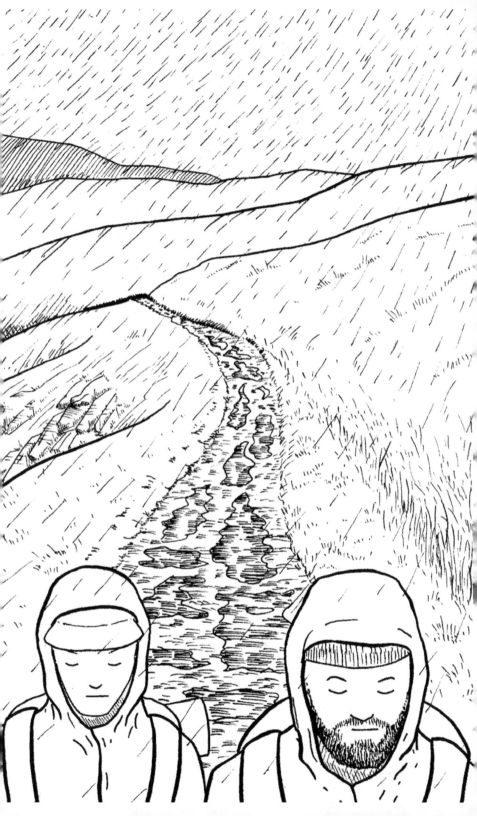

When we were left on our own, I slowly started to open my pack. There was a puddle of water at the bottom. I pulled out my collection of zipper-lock and "waterproof" bags that were supposed to keep my gear and food dry, but everything was wet. I started to cry. I didn't have any dry clothes, I was cold and wet, and my down sleeping bag was compressed and dripping with water, which meant it wouldn't keep me warm.

I started shivering. Brew's sleeping bag was damp, but much drier than my own. He instructed me to take off my wet clothes and crawl inside. He then laid down beside me and started rubbing my back with his hand to try and warm me up faster. I looked up at him sitting beside me.

"Are you going to quit?" I asked.

"No way," he replied. "I don't care if it rains like this for the next ten days. I've given too much to this trail to give up now," he said.

That night, lying on the cold dirt floor of a barn that must have been several hundred years old, I had two revelations. The first concerned the Virgin Mary. I had heard the Christmas story dozens of times, and I had even played a shepherd in a church pageant, but I don't think I had ever stopped to think about how Mary must have felt going into labor with Jesus. That night, it occurred to me that if I had been in Mary's shoes and had known that God had the power to create a divine conception, yet had overlooked a reservation at the inn, I would have been pretty frustrated.

Second, I decided that I really did want to go back and try for the overall record on the Appalachian Trail. I had given too much to that trail to give up now.

I was wrong when I thought that it would be difficult to convince Brew to return to the Appalachian Trail. By the end of our

European hiking trip, we both had committed to attempting the overall record the following summer.

After having almost a year to think it through, Brew said that he would support me in whatever decision I made. On the same note, he made it very clear that if it was up to him, he would not choose to go back to the trail and run support because it is difficult, because there is a lot of pressure that goes along with it, and because it is not the most relaxing way to spend his summer vacation. But, he said, if it was important to me, then he would be fully supportive.

I was thankful that Brew was so honest and realistic about his participation. Unlike 2008, this time my husband knew exactly what he was agreeing to. That transparency gave me the confidence to look him in the eyes and reply, "It's important to me. It's really important to me."

After we made our decision, we started to tell other people about it. At first, it went well. I told Warren and Horton that I wanted to try for the overall record, and they not only thought I had a chance at succeeding, but they both agreed to help me in the endeavor. Then I wrote a lengthy email to Andrew Thompson, who was still the overall record holder. He responded graciously and with encouragement, offering to provide any of the daily mileages from his record and saying he would try to come out and hike with me when I passed through New Hampshire. However, after those three interactions, the responses became increasingly negative.

My mom argued that I would wreck my body and not be able to have children. I had close friends who said I would tarnish my women's record if I failed in an attempt for the overall record. And the majority of the hiking and trail running community thought that I was conceited or delusional for thinking I could break a record that had been held by elite male trail runners for the past thirty years.

Some of the online hiking and running forums that I belonged to began to show a flurry of unkind comments in response to my announcement. Most of the runners thought I didn't have the ability to set the record, and most of the hikers thought that wanting to set the record meant that I didn't truly appreciate or respect the trail. At first I was upset at all the negative feedback, and then Brew offered a simple answer: "Ignore it."

For seven months leading up to my hike, I didn't read or access any website or news source that offered commentary on my hike. Shutting out most of the external voices made it a lot easier to listen to my heart. I also had a lengthy sit-down visit with my doctor to talk about the long-term physical ramifications of hiking forty-six miles per day for a month and a half. Her underwhelmed response helped assuage my mother's fears.

Occasionally, I still had to deal with reporters who called and asked me about my upcoming hike. I was amazed at how every interview focused on a fear of failure. Reporters wanted to talk more about not setting a record than about actually accomplishing my goal. It made me realize how much our culture is paralyzed by the fear of losing. I wasn't worried about not succeeding; I was worried about not trying.

In a worst-case scenario, I was going to spend some quality time on a trail that I love, with the man I love, doing what I love. I didn't see what was so scary about that.

I was scared about how difficult it would be, and how much I would hurt, but I wasn't afraid of letting other people down. I loved hiking. I loved the trails. But at the end of the day, my self-worth wasn't tied to the trail. I believed that God loved me unconditionally, and I knew that my relationships with my husband, family, and friends were not performance based.

As the time drew near, instead of being filled with anxiety, I was overcome with peace. I knew that just by starting the trail, I would never have to look back and wonder *what if.*

I decided that, if nothing else, the training had made the decision worthwhile. The benefit of having my own hiking company was that I was able to spend fifteen to twenty-five hours a week on the trail in the three months leading up to the summer. When I was not guiding, but rather training on my own, I tried to find the steepest mountains near my house and go up them as many times as possible.

One morning I woke up, walked out my front door, and hiked forty miles to the top of Mount Mitchell, the same peak where Brew and I had enjoyed one of our first dates. On my twenty-eighth birthday, I pulled another forty-mile day hiking almost entirely uphill from the French Broad River to Black Balsam on the Mountains-to-Sea Trail. Brew met me with pizza and beer at the finish, which made it a perfect day.

Because I knew the summer would not allow time for scenic rest stops, I indulged myself during training by always carrying a camera and taking breaks at waterfalls and overlooks to enjoy the view. Sometimes, after a long day of training, I would hesitate before taking a shower, thinking that perhaps I should go ahead and train my mind and body to get used to the discomfort and dirt that I would encounter that summer. But I almost always succumbed to a warm rinse and a full eight hours of rest—I figured that I should make the most of it while I still could.

6

A ROCKY START

EARLY JUNE 2011—JUNE 21, 2011

Nothing felt strange about leaving home in early June to drive up to Maine and start the trail. For the past eight years, I had spent the summers hiking. The well-refined tasks of packing, wrapping up work, and cleaning up our house for a renter filled our thoughts and our time before the departure.

Upon leaving Asheville, we enjoyed our two-and-a-half-day road trip up to northern New England. Brew had a bounce in his step that I hadn't seen in a while. Not only was he excited to conclude a very trying school year, but he was also recovering nicely from the ACL surgery that he had undergone in March. Because of his unexpected knee injury, he would not be able to hike with me this summer. But thankfully, many of our friends offered their on-trail and off-trail support as a substitute.

It was a bit demoralizing to parallel almost the entire 2,000+ mile A.T. in less than three days especially when I knew how difficult it would be to work my way back down south on foot. But the full magnitude of the undertaking did not set in until we met Warren and Melissa in the small logging town of Millinocket, Maine, the closest civilization to Katahdin.

Warren had offered to help us with road support and logistics on the first two weeks of the trip. Melissa was a friend from home who had joined the team once Brew sustained his injury. She offered to help us by taking photographs, doing crew chores, and providing me with some much-needed company on the trail.

Together, we sat around a table at the A.T. Café in Millinocket. The four of us went over the details of the first twelve days. I knew the first two weeks on the trail would be the most difficult. I would be traveling over the most challenging terrain, and my body would be going through all the aches, pains, and adjustments of a multi-day hike. There was limited crew access on many sections, which meant I would be traveling long stretches on my own and without resupply. The weather was also a major factor in this portion of the trail. The tall peaks in Maine and the White Mountains of New Hampshire threatened snow, sleet, and violent thundershowers, even throughout the summer. Being in the wrong spot during a bad storm in this terrain could not only mean the end of my record, it could also be life-threatening.

Warren had planned out a very ambitious schedule for the first two states, and I had agreed to it. I decided that the sooner I could make it through Maine and New Hampshire, the better.

As far as Warren was concerned, there was another reason I needed to accomplish high miles in the beginning of the hike.

"Once you get past the Mason-Dixon Line, you won't be able to match Andrew Thompson day for day, so it's important to establish a lead in the first half of the hike."

"How do you know I can't match Andy in the southeast?!" I fired back.

"Well, I'm glad that you *think* you can," Warren said with a smirk. "Just remember, once Andrew hit Maryland, he put in consistent fifty-mile days until the finish. If you fall behind before the half-way point, it will be oppressive knowing that you will have to average over fifty miles a day to break the men's record."

I corrected him. "You mean the *overall* record."

"What?" Warren didn't understand what I was getting at.

"You mean the *overall* record, not the men's record."

I wasn't trying to be disagreeable. The fact was, I wasn't trying to beat the men's record. I didn't have anything against the boys. But by phrasing it that way, I was already considered an outsider, an underdog. The world may have seen me as a dark horse, but I didn't see myself that way. The "overall record" sounded far more inclusive. Wording was important and would continue to be important throughout the hike.

The next forty-seven days would be filled with concise mantras and encouraging self-talk. Whether it stemmed from sports psychology or the insanity of spending long periods of time alone, I do not know. But I was certain that I would draw from my favorite phrases of hikes past, such as "Every step is one step closer," "Hike it out," and "It can't always get worse." I also knew that there would be new phrases that summer, and one that had already surfaced was, "I belong."

I belonged out on the trail, and I belonged among the other A.T. record holders. Just because no woman had ever tried for the record or set the record in the past didn't mean that I hadn't earned the right to be at the base of Katahdin, ready to establish a new mark. This wasn't about being male or female; this was about being the best. And I believed that my best was good enough for the *overall* record.

The next day was spitting rain, but I had waited two full years for this moment, and I didn't want to delay any longer. We drove to Baxter State Park and established our campsite at the base of Katahdin. I spent the rest of the day making sure that the car was organized, knowing that Brew would quickly undo all my hard work. But when the chores were over and all the gear, food, and first aid had been put in its proper place, I still looked for something else—anything else—to do.

I found myself feeling both anxious and impatient. The waning hours of the day felt endless, and the sun seemed locked in the sky. Knowing that my miles would be slower through the technical terrain in New England, we had decided to start the hike close to the summer equinox in order to maximize the daylight hours. I never looked forward to night hiking, but on the rock scrambles and steep inclines of Maine and New Hampshire, I dreaded it.

At 9:45 p.m., when the darkness settled on the forest, I had the excuse I needed to crawl into my tent. I zipped up my sleeping bag, then stared wide-eyed at the thin gray fabric of the ceiling. The moon was so bright that it looked like someone was shining a flashlight outside. Every fifteen minutes, I checked my wristwatch, hoping more time had passed than I'd expected. Even though I knew that my watch alarm was set for sometime just after midnight, it was still my longest night of the entire trip.

Finally when the piercing sound of the alarm filled the night air, I slipped on my shoes and a jacket and broke out of the tent like a caged animal. I wanted to start extra early on the first day since my initial miles did not count toward my summer total. I needed to reach the summit and touch the sign for the record attempt to begin.

I started my ascent up the Greatest Mountain. I had completed this hike as a recent college grad and as a recent newlywed. Now I was here because I needed to know what I was capable of. My mind was racing. The third time on the trail would be the charm, I told myself. Either that, or a sign of insanity. Either way, I would need both luck and a little bit of madness to be successful this summer.

As I reached the end of the rock scramble, I looked out across the tableland that leads to the mountain summit. I turned off my headlamp. It was 3:25 a.m. The full moon illuminated large cairns that marked the trail. The gleam was so bright that I no longer needed artificial light to guide me down the path.

My feet gracefully carried me over the loose stones and dirt of the ridge. My breathing was short and quick, and my heart felt like it wanted to escape from inside my jacket.

The path began to rise to the summit. And then it appeared, the beautiful haunting sign that marks the northern terminus of the trail. I slowed to a reverent pace as I neared the worn brown marker. I approached the wooden altar that demanded so much sacrifice, and I stood before it. I reached out my right hand and began to trace the large white letters. *K-A-T-A-H-D-I-N*.

I took the deepest, most relaxing breath that I had enjoyed since starting my ascent of the mountain. I looked up at the moon watching over me and experienced a penetrating sense of calm. Part of my burden was already lifting. I would not have to wonder *what might have been*. I would never have to think about *what if.* The answers were out there. Now all I had to do was hike to them.

Every ounce of me loved being back on the trail. I felt graceful and fluid as I moved through the woods. Even though I had hiked on six continents, I still preferred the Appalachian Mountains.

Every time I set foot on the A.T., I feel like it is giving me a loving embrace. The stifling humidity in the south is like a warm breath on my neck, the verdant tunnel through the forest like long, strong arms enveloping me. The wisdom of the ancient summits whispers in my ear, and the consistency of the wildlife and plant life is like a familiar scent. I welcome the embrace, and it does not let me go.

I enjoyed the blue skies that welcomed me on the first day of the journey. I knew that they wouldn't last, but I was grateful to at least start in good weather. Based on previous experience, I was also prepared for many of the obstacles that the trail threw my way. I knew to take only one hiking stick to the top of Katahdin, because I would need my free hand to help with rock scrambles on the descent. I was covered in all-natural bug spray to keep the black flies at bay, and I carried a pair of dry socks to change into after my two early-morning river crossings.

And as familiar as it all felt, I was struck by the subtle differences that made this a completely new experience. The water in the rivers was higher than it had been in the past, the reflection of Katahdin in Rainbow Lake was more brilliant, and I saw fewer people and stepped in more mud than I did in either 2005 or 2008. It was both exciting and daunting to know that no matter how many times I covered the distance of the A.T., I would never hike the same trail twice.

I met my crew four times that afternoon, which meant my pack stayed light and so did my heart. I loved seeing Brew's smiling face and hearing Melissa clapping when I came to a road crossing. Each time I arrived, they would pull out a folding chair and ask what food and drinks I wanted from the car. They refilled my daypack, and once or twice, Brew even rubbed bug spray on my legs so that I wouldn't have to.

It was amazing how quickly I got used to this treatment.

At the final road crossing of the day, I exited the woods without fanfare or greeting to find Melissa and Brew sleeping under bug netting and Warren nowhere in sight. I was disappointed and a little frustrated. I knew that the entire team had been up since three a.m., but if I was still going, then I expected the same from the crew. I grabbed some snacks and replenished my water bottles on my own at the car, and then I shut the trunk door loudly to wake up Melissa and Brew. They both bolted upright and looked at each other in horror. I could tell by the look in their eyes, the apologies, and the offers to help, that they felt horrible for lying down on the job, but by the time they were on their feet, I was already ten yards down the trail.

After shoving a handful of cheddar cheese and pretzels in my mouth and drinking some juice, it occurred to me that, like clockwork, I had become irrational. I had covered over forty miles, it was after five p.m., and I no longer had any perspective. As I began to digest the calories, I realized that I should be thankful that my husband and friends were out here helping me, not upset that they were exhausted and needed a quick nap. I realized once again why this was so hard on Brew. And I recognized that I would need to do a better job of controlling the hungry, tired monster that came out around six p.m.

That night when I arrived at our campsite, I walked out of the woods apologetic and appreciative. Warren and Melissa had already set up their tents and retired. Brew had our tent set up as well, and my freeze-dried dinner was cooked and waiting for me. Inside our shelter, Brew hunted the dozen or so black flies that had made their way in. This from the man who had scowled at me on our first date when I squished an ant because it was enjoying the picnic I had packed. He hated cruelty—even toward insects. But that was before 2008, when he was introduced to the black flies in Maine. Now he made it a point to kill as many of the tiny blood-sucking insects as possible.

On my side of the tent, I was using a handful of wet wipes to try to remove the grime and dirt that already covered my body. It was hard to believe that three nights ago, we had stayed in a hotel with a hot shower, an indoor pool, and a clean king-sized bed. Now, I was scrubbing my body down with a product primarily intended for babies' bottoms, listening to my husband verbally abuse tiny biting insects while he randomly clapped his hands in the air in an effort to squash them. It was both comforting and horrifying to consider that this would be our routine for the next month and a half.

The next two days were exactly what I expected. They were hard.

I was sore and in pain, but I was still incredibly happy to be back on the trail. Because I had traveled this terrain twice before, it seemed like every new turn held an old memory. It was amazing how much of the trail I actually remembered. Sometimes I would reach out for a limb on a steep climb and remember placing my hand there before. Other times, when I stepped on a wooden bog log that protected the fragile lowlands, I would recall slipping and falling on that same damp piece of wood three years prior.

The one thing I didn't remember with such clarity was just how arduous the Appalachian Trail was. No matter how many times I told myself that hiking would be challenging and tedious, I was never fully prepared.

The A.T. is not a smooth, well-graded trail. It is rugged, steep, and filled with constant elevation change. There are fallen trees that you must climb over and crawl under, river crossings that saturate your lower half and threaten to whisk you downstream, and sections of mud that seem to take pleasure in swallowing your ankles.

It is a blessing and a curse not to fully remember the challenges. This selective memory allowed me to return to the trail, but it also caused me to second-guess my decision and my abilities once I arrived.

Although the Hundred-Mile Wilderness is less difficult than some sections of trail in western Maine and New Hampshire, it has two very challenging mountain ranges. The north side of Whitecap leaves you feeling as if you are condemned to a never-ending staircase. And the steep grade of the Barren Chairback Mountains makes you feel as if you are scrambling up a ladder, not a mountain. I had to climb both ascents in one day, and the task left me both exhausted and elated.

When I arrived at Long Pond Stream at the west end of the Barren Chairback range, it was dusk. I quickly went down to the river to bathe, but as I approached it, I placed my foot on a slick rock and fell forward, my hands and knees landing in the water. I pulled myself back to the shore and grabbed my ankle. Something didn't feel right, so I gently tried to roll it clockwise and I knew immediately that it was sprained. I could still put pressure on it and I was thankful that it wasn't injured worse, because I knew that I could keep hiking on a sprained ankle. But I hated feeling like I had come so far that day only to sustain a setback when I had *finished* hiking.

I submerged my ankle in the cold water to reduce the swelling. Sitting there in the dark, on the banks of Long Pond Stream, with my elbows on my knees and my face buried in my hands, I knew that all summer, I would feel as if I were hiking two steps forward and one step back. And I was humbly reminded that it would only take one split second, one misstep, or one mistake to end my dream.

The next day, my ankle hurt and my energy level was depleted, but I was still happy to be on the trail. I didn't make it quite as far as I wanted to by the end of the day, but I knew I had set myself up to cross the Kennebec River the following morning.

The Kennebec is a wide, raging river that flows near the small town of Caratunk, Maine. Historically, many thru-hikers crossed it on foot. Then after someone lost their life in the ford, the

Appalachian Trail Conservancy implemented a canoe ferry for hikers. On my last two thru-hikes, I had taken the ferry across. But this time I wanted to try to ford the river.

It had nothing to do with the record. In fact, fording would exert far more energy than just riding across in a canoe. And timing-wise, there was no real advantage since I'd arrived at the water's edge just before the ferryman started to take hikers across. It was just that I had always wanted to cross the river on foot.

I loved listening to stories of thru-hikers from the sixties and seventies who said crossing the Kennebec was almost as meaningful to them as climbing Katahdin. I was out here to experience the trail in a new and different way, and because I wasn't traveling with a full pack on my shoulders, I thought this would be the perfect time to ford. Plus, I had Warren.

Warren had completed dozens of successful fords across the Kennebec. He knew that the best place to ford was a quarter mile upstream from where the canoe crossed. He knew where the sandbars were in the middle of the river. And he knew by the ripples on the water whether or not it was safe to cross. The Kennebec is a dam-controlled river, so the water level varies greatly depending on the hour and day. The morning that I came to the Kennebec, the river was raging, and Warren said we needed to wait.

So I used the next hour to consume as many calories as possible and to clean the scrapes and blisters that I had collected over the past three days. I knew that if the water levels did not decrease, I would end up taking the canoe ferry across the river for a third time. But after about ninety minutes, Warren came back from the Kennebec and said that it would be challenging, but that he felt we could make it across safely.

As I put all my belongings in a plastic bag in my daypack, Warren talked me through what to do if I lost my footing and the current pushed me downstream. We talked about my body position in the water, how to hold my legs if I was swept away, and—worst-case scenario—how to swim like hell back to shore. It wasn't much of a pep talk.

I quickly walked down to the official canoe crossing to make sure I didn't skip even a small portion of the "official" A.T., then I backtracked to find Warren waiting and wading upstream. He was already in ankle-deep, ready to go.

I placed my shoes in the cold, rushing water beside him, and together we took one step at a time deeper into the river. I couldn't believe how fast the water was moving. I was using my hiking poles to help me, but every time I tried to place one into the water, the current swept it away before it touched the riverbed. The crossing was manageable when the water was knee-deep or lower, but as soon as I was in thigh-deep, I had trouble keeping my feet beneath my body. In a split second, the river really could wash me downstream. Warren was slightly ahead of me, and I tried to stay behind him at an angle so his round belly would act as an eddy and diffuse the current.

The entire time we were struggling across, Warren said over and over again, "Feet down." He said it rhythmically, almost like a chant. "Feet down. Feet down. Feet down." I appreciated the repetitive instruction and comfort of knowing that Warren was nearby.

After progressing roughly twenty yards, I found myself sports-bra deep in the current. I couldn't plant my feet, and my toes just grazed the rocks below before being forced downstream. The most important thing I could do was keep myself vertical and upright. Every muscle in my body was tense and I tried desperately to stay anchored to the river bottom. Even though I couldn't get a solid foothold on the slick rocks beneath me, I needed to keep my toes touching the earth. If I bent my knee too much or flexed my hips, I would be swept away.

When I was still sports-bra deep, I watched Warren rise out of the river before me. We weren't even a third of the way across, but suddenly the water became increasingly shallow. We had reached

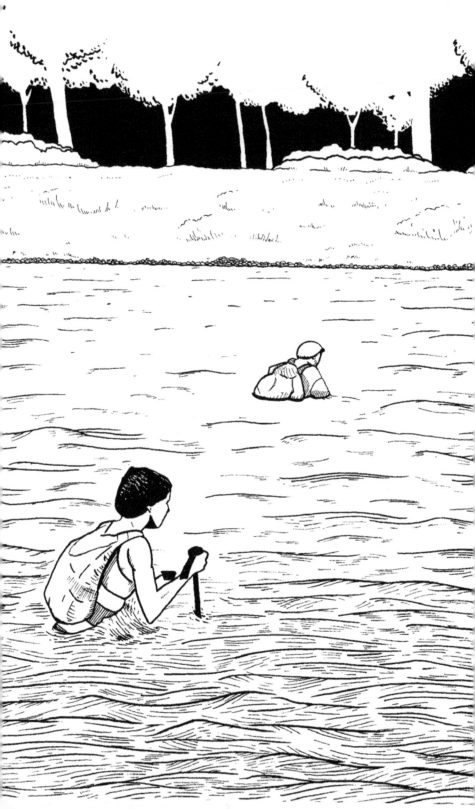

the first sandbar. After struggling so hard for the past few minutes, it was shocking to be knee-deep and comfortably, carefully
making progress once again.

Warren looked back at me, "Rest here. We have to go through
another channel in the middle of the river. After that, we'll have
one more sandbar to catch our breath, and then we will cross the
third channel."

Third channel?! No wonder crossing the Kennebec was so difficult. It wasn't like you were crossing one river; it was like you
were crossing three.

I didn't respond verbally to Warren; instead, I nodded in understanding. I was too scared and focused to say anything.

After two or three minutes of rest, we started our journey
through the second channel. It was just as difficult as the first one,
but every time Warren repeated "feet down," I tried to keep my
shoes on the bottom of the river and move them a little closer to
the opposite shore.

When we made it to the second sandbar, I looked back. Brew
and Melissa were both sitting there looking at us, but they seemed
so small. I couldn't believe how far we had come and how wide the
river really was—or that we still had our last leg to travel.

Thankfully, the final channel of water came only to my waist,
and twenty minutes after we had started, Warren and I arrived at
the west bank of the river. I looked back at Brew and raised my
hands into the air in celebration. The river was wild and free, and
that was exactly how I felt, too.

Our successful ford of the Kennebec gave me a surge of confidence that kept me hiking strong throughout the rest of the day.
In the late afternoon, I was making my way up Bigelow Mountain
when I came across a northbound thru-hiker.

At this point, I had already seen four or five of them. It was still mid-June, and these folks were only days away from the end of their journeys. That meant most of them had completed the trek in only three months. The majority of thru-hikers take four to six months, but with high-calorie diets and lightweight gear, efficient hikers who don't spend a lot of time (and money) in towns can finish the trail in less than one hundred days.

The first handful of thru-hikers in the 1950s and 1960s usually completed the trek in about four months as well. However, in the 1960s there were not as many hiker hostels, shuttles, or local amenities for the trail community. These services are usually perceived as aids for a hiker on his journey—and they are. But they can also be a distraction.

Watching this thru-hiker descend toward me, it was clear that he was not easily distracted. This man was short and wiry. He appeared to be in his fifties, but he moved like he was in his twenties. His clothes were brown and smudged, and he wore a lightweight pack with homemade modifications. Even when he was close enough to me that I could detect a distinct thru-hiker smell, he still kept his head ducked and his eyes focused on the trail.

When he was finally at arm's reach, he lifted his head so I could see his entire face, or at least the part that wasn't hidden under his scraggily copper-toned beard.

Immediately, he exclaimed, "Odyssa!"

"Yes?" I responded hesitantly.

"It's me, Rambler. I was wondering when I would see you. Here, let me give you some of my food."

Rambler reached into the side pocket on his pack and pulled out a bottle of Powerade, then he dug into the front pouch to search for a Little Debbie Cosmic brownie. If his appearance had not given him away, the lightweight, high-calorie, processed brownie that he produced from his pack was enough to convince me that he was a thru-hiker. Rambler held out his offering, and I gladly accepted.

Although he was dirtier and hairier than the last time we met, I now remembered him vividly. I recalled discussing his love of Cosmic brownies—which have a shelf life of several years—at a hiker convention this past winter. We had agreed it was shocking that snacks so completely void of nutritional content tasted so good on a long hike.

I also remembered this short, fit man with a cap and spectacles because, like me, Rambler was a repeat offender. He had hiked the A.T. multiple times. He was also a Triple Crowner, which meant he had completed not only the A.T. but he had also hiked the 2,665-mile Pacific Crest Trail and the 3,100-mile Continental Divide Trail.

I was excited to see a friendly face and I was thankful for the excuse to take a quick rest. But while I gladly stopped to talk to Rambler (and accept his snacks), he didn't let me have a sustained break.

"Are you trying to make it to the next road? You still have over ten miles to go. You better keep hiking so you don't get stuck scrambling down the backside of the Bigelows in the dark."

Unfortunately, he was right. I had some really tricky footing coming up, and I needed to push hard to make it through the ankle-twisting terrain before dark. I nodded to Rambler in agreement and thanked him for the brownie and then I kept hiking. As I scrambled up the next rocky incline, Rambler called after me. "You're doing great! If you need any help when you get to Pennsylvania, send me an email. I'll be done with the trail and back home when you get there."

I knew that I wouldn't need Rambler's help in Pennsylvania. I had dialed in my support crew months before, but seeing him in the middle of the Maine backcountry—a familiar face and an unexpected encouragement—allowed me to pick up the pace and make it over the Bigelows without the help of a headlamp.

On day five, I woke up to a chill in the air and a cold, runny nose. There are some hikers out there who consider temperatures below fifty degrees perfect for hiking. I am not one of those hikers.

Crawling out of my sleeping bag, my muscles felt stiffer than usual. After a quick bite to eat, I immediately started to hike. I knew the quickest way to get warm was to move. The problem was that the trail made a 1,500-foot climb. And the higher I hiked, the colder I felt. The wind started whipping through the trees near the summit, and I came off the back of the mountain with my jaw clenched to keep my teeth from chattering.

When I reached the next road, I met my crew, put on more clothes, and tried to eat a lot more food. I had been eating every hour, but I was still starving. My body felt like it wanted an extra layer of fat to combat the crisp weather.

In the next section, I had two difficult river crossings. The fords weren't as wide or as treacherous as the Kennebec, but because it had stormed during the night, the rivers were swollen and moving very fast. I couldn't make out any of the rocks beneath the torrents. So deciding where to put my feet proved to be a cold, wet trial-and-error process.

At the first river ford, there was a loose wooden plank that allowed hikers to avoid the worst of the rapids. The problem was that the water level was the same height as the board, and the wood was slick and wet.

If I had stopped long enough to think about it, I probably would have realized that walking on a beam partially submerged by a raging current wasn't safe. But I committed to the act before considering all my options. And it wasn't until I was halfway across the board that I was overcome with fear. I looked up at the water around me. Fallen tree limbs and debris raced past my feet.

My legs suddenly stopped moving. I regretted taking the risk. Instead of just getting wet in a ford, I now risked falling hard into the water and onto the unseen rocks below the surface.

Fear is supposed to be a protective instinct, so I don't know why it causes every muscle in your body to tense up and stop working. My sudden inhibition left me momentarily paralyzed and made it even more difficult to cross the now-submerged four-inch walkway. I took a deep breath and then willed my feet to slide across the last few yards of the board. When I made it safely to the other side, I thanked God for keeping me safe and silently vowed to him—and to my mother—that I would not be as reckless in the future.

At the next river crossing, I plowed straight through and arrived safely at the other side.

Exiting the waist-deep rapids, my legs felt even more stiff and tense than they had that morning. Because of the chill in the air, the freezing water, and my fear, I never felt like my muscles had the opportunity to warm up and stretch out as they normally would. Or perhaps they were just sore and inflexible after covering one-hundred and eighty-eight miles in the past four days. I couldn't pinpoint the primary reason for it; all I knew is that my legs felt like fossilized tree trunks.

At least I was about to start ascending Saddleback Mountain. That would loosen up my limbs. Saddleback is a monster climb from both directions, and I liked it. There are lots of rocks and roots to pull up on, so at times it is almost like climbing a stepladder—a stepladder that leads to one of best views on the entire trail.

This is the same stretch of trail where Brew and I had missed a resupply in 2008, and I'd had to survive the climb by eating a package of Chips Ahoy cookies given to me by a thru-hiker. But on that hike, a view from the top of the mountain had made it easy to forget about the climb and the struggle that had gotten me there. It had even made it easy to forget about the women's trail record and my husband waiting patiently at the next road.

I expected an incredible view and a transcendent moment at the end of this climb, too. A moment where everything felt right.

Instead, I arrived at the exposed ridge leading to the summit and the strong, bitter wind took my breath away. It also made hiking out in the open three times more difficult than walking in the woods and made my fingers, wrists, and face feel like ice. I knew that the frigid conditions and my added exertion meant I needed to get off the ridge as soon as possible. So I decided to run until I could return to tree cover and escape the wind. I ducked my head and focused on the trail. I tried to look up at times to see the incredible view, but I could keep my eyes open for only a few seconds before the piercing wind filled them with tears.

After I crested the mountain, I was able to increase my pace. I had been on exposed granite for several miles, and all of a sudden, I started to feel a pain in my lower right shin. I put more weight on the left side of my body to provide some relief, but then I felt a sharp discomfort in that leg, as well. Both my shins hurt, but I knew the pain would go away when I could make it to tree cover and stop running.

I entered the forest and began hiking, but the pain in my legs remained. In fact, it actually seemed to be getting worse. I treaded slowly and carefully down the mountain, but still the tenderness intensified. Whenever my toe caught a root or rock, the agony was too great to keep inside, and I released an involuntarily wail.

It felt like I would never get to the next road. The section felt infinitely longer than on my previous two hikes. I began to wonder whether they had rerouted and extended this portion of the trail. Finally, I came to a stream with a wooden bridge. I didn't understand why the local trail maintainers chose to build a small wooden bridge over a simple creek when they left the raging rivers untouched.

On the opposite side, I saw a note left by my husband. He had spelled out the word "LOVE" with broken sticks and branches. Because of the note, I knew that I must be within a quarter mile of the road; Brew couldn't hike any farther than that since he was still recovering from ACL surgery. It should have been a physical relief to know that I was so close to the road, but now that I knew I was nearing a respite, I stopped trying to repress my feelings. As I walked across the bridge, pain spread through every inch of my body and tears slid down my cheeks. All I wanted to do was get to Brew and get off of my feet.

When I arrived at Route 4, I fell into Brew's arms and he helped me to the car where I could sit and elevate my legs. I had put in thirty-three miles since five a.m., the sun was starting to set, and my final destination for the day was a road ten miles away. I felt horrible all over, and my shins were screaming. There was no way I could hike another ten miles.

"Don't sit too long. You need to keep going to make it to the next road," Warren said.

The past few days, I had felt like Warren was trying to push me farther than my body was willing to go.

"I can't make it tonight. My legs have never hurt this badly. And I don't want to night hike until midnight," I said.

Warren countered, "That will make the schedule for the next few days very difficult." Then he sat down in his car where he could stare at the numbers on his proposed itinerary.

I knew Warren was right, but I didn't want to hear it. The road crossings in Maine and New Hampshire were spread out. If I fell off-schedule, it would mean several nights spent on the trail without the help of my crew or my husband's company.

The ideal scenario was to end every day at a road crossing. I knew that there would be some days when I would need to spend the night on the trail because of mileage and accessibility. That was fine. I had no problem backpacking or spending a night in the woods.

But carrying a full pack was extra work and it was inefficient. Even if Melissa or another friend could come with me and share some of the weight, it would still take more time and energy than moving through the forest with a daypack. And this record was all about saving time and energy.

But in that moment, I wasn't able to think about logistics, efficiency, or my long-term schedule. All I knew was that I was in pain and I wanted to be with the man who left me eco-notes in the middle of the trail.

I was busy washing down the maximum prescribed dose of ibuprofen with a full pint of Ben and Jerry's ice cream when Warren came back to our car.

"You need to keep going," he said.

I was beginning to feel frustrated and hurt by Warren's constant prodding.

"Warren, there is *no way* that I can make it to the next road," I protested.

"You don't have to," he replied. "You can either put on a backpack and hike in with Melissa to camp in another three or four miles. Or, if you think you can hike six miles, then Brew and I can meet you on the trail."

I hadn't done the trail sixteen times like Warren, but I had done it enough to know there was not a road in the middle of this section.

"How are you going to get there?" I asked.

"I know a way that's not on the map."

"And Brew can walk there with his knee?"

"Yes. We'll have your tent set up when you arrive."

In another five minutes, I was back on the trail, and Melissa was keeping me company. I didn't feel like *I* had made the choice to continue hiking, but I knew it was the best decision.

I made sure to leave the car with two hiking sticks in my hands for the last stretch. I loved hiking with poles to help keep pressure off my joints and to aid me in climbing up the mountains. But most of the time in Maine, I left them in the car or only took one because I needed to have my hands available to grab the rocks and roots while scrambling. At this point, though, I needed my sticks. They were no longer hiking poles; they were crutches.

Melissa and I began our hike, and at first I thought my legs felt a little better. But within ten minutes, the same pain that I had felt on Saddleback had returned, and after an hour my legs felt even more inflamed and aggravated than before.

Melissa and I both love the trail, and we did a lot of hiking together in the mountains of North Carolina. On most of our hikes, we spent hours talking about the wonders of nature. In the first few days of our record, she had hiked several miles with me each day. And during those stretches, it was great to hear her talk about how awesome it was to be in the woods, and how amazing the forests in Maine were, and how free she felt on the trail.

But tonight, Melissa hiked fifteen feet in front of me, rambling on about how perfect everything was. The only time she paused was when I stubbed my toe and yelled curse words to the sky. I think she was gushing positive comments and romantic rhetoric to try to motivate me and make me remember how much I loved hiking. But it didn't work. So now, not only were my legs bothering me, but Melissa was, too.

I do love to hike. Melissa didn't have to remind me of how I felt about the trail. That was understood. But what *she* didn't understand was how much pain I was in. And when you are consumed with hurt, the last thing you want to hear is someone telling you how wonderful everything is.

I had warned Melissa when she volunteered to help that it wasn't always going to be fun or easy. I also told her that there would be times on the trail when I would be highly unpleasant to be around, and I didn't want her to come if she thought it would affect our friendship off the trail. She was not deterred. Before today, I had been nice. But now I was hurting too badly to be anything but honest.

"Do you hear those sounds? I love listening to the insects at night. And look, you can see the last tiny speck of the sun setting over the horizon. Isn't it beautiful?"

"Melissa," I said curtly, "it's really hard for me to hear about how great everything is when I am in so much pain."

There was a pause. I could tell she was not expecting criticism. And I didn't want to give it, but I was suffering too much not to say something.

"Okay," she said. Then she hiked a little farther in front of me.

I couldn't tell whether or not I had hurt her feelings. But I also couldn't spend any time thinking about it. The pain was too consuming.

After an hour of hiking with my headlamp, watching Melissa's beam weave in and out of the trees farther up the trail, I heard male voices. It was Brew and Warren!

I was glad to be done for the day, and I was really glad to be with my husband. I crawled into the tent, forced down some dinner, then cuddled up next to him. He started to say our evening prayer, but I wasn't paying attention. I was so tired. It was hard to focus, hard to move, and hard to keep my eyelids open. It even felt hard to breathe.

That night, I did something I have never done before. I snored. I must have snored loudly and for most of the night, because Melissa said she heard it from her tent thirty feet away. But Brew never woke me up, and he never complained. The next morning, he helped me get ready, then packed up all of our gear and hiked back to the nearest road, where he got in the car and drove around to meet me later that morning.

All day, I felt horrible. At my first road crossing, Warren was there to meet me. He had some duct tape in his car and I wrapped my shins with it to try and alleviate the pain, but it didn't work.

At the next road crossing there was a river, and instead of taking a break near the car, I stopped at the water to submerge my red, swollen shins. Brew gave me medicine and athletic tape to rewrap my legs.

Melissa hiked with me on the next stretch, which was a huge help. She was relatively quiet. I assumed she didn't know what to say to make it better. But her presence and staring down at the back of her shoes helped take my mind off the discomfort.

Melissa continued with me to the base of Baldpate Mountain, where I once again set out on my own. Swollen flesh sat on top of the white athletic tape that surrounded my shins. I had dealt with the shin splints long enough at this point to realize that they were painful going uphill, more painful on level ground, and most painful going down. Above all, catching my toe on a root or rock was unbearable.

After concentrating on every step and trying with all my might not to graze the obstacles strewn along the footpath, I reached the exposed apex of Baldpate Mountain. Once there, I turned my body and walked backward down the steep slope since hiking backward didn't hurt quite as much as hiking forward.

Once I made it past the sheerest section on the descent, I noticed Warren hiking in front of me. So far, the only portion of the trail we had traveled together was the Kennebec River. However, he had wanted to hike this segment to work on his current section hike that, when complete, would mark his seventeenth completion of the trail.

"How far do we have to go?" I called out.

"It's two more miles until we reach the road."

That was all we said. I was in too much pain to have a conversation. I walked in front of Warren and within minutes, the sun set and we pulled out our headlamps. Something felt symbolic about the encroaching darkness. I felt like I had lost hope, and everything started to feel worse. I began to cry. Warren still didn't say anything.

I screamed every time my legs were jolted by the unexpected impact of a fallen branch or stone littering the trail. Usually, when I cried on the trail, it had at least a little to do with fatigue or hunger. But even though I was at the end of a long day, that night my tears were entirely caused by pain. In twenty-eight years, I had experienced many illnesses, injuries, and a broken bone, but I had never hurt this badly.

Roads can be deceptive. I heard the road at Grafton Notch about a mile before the trail crossed the highway. And because I could hear the constant purr of passenger vehicles and the loud roar of semi-trucks, I thought my agony was almost over. But it wasn't. I kept stumbling along, shrieking and crying, with no end in sight. I felt like the mythical Greek figure Tantalus, faced with the eternal punishment of being almost within reach of his heart's desire yet not being able to obtain it.

Finally, I saw a light through the trees. It was Brew standing at the trailhead with a headlamp. My crying turned to sobs as I fell into his arms. He held me for several minutes without saying anything.

Finally, when my gasping breaths relaxed a bit, he took my hand and started to lead me across the road. As soon as my feet hit the pavement, I began to sob again. The pain was consuming. I reached the other side and fell to my knees. Then I crawled the next thirty feet to reach our tent in the forest. I had said that I would not quit this hike, that I would hike until I had to crawl. But there I was, on day six, already crawling.

That night in our tent, I continued to sniffle and cry while trying to choke down a freeze-dried mac and cheese dinner. I had my legs propped up with ice on my shins. The slightest movement hurt. The worst pain was in my legs, but the sensation was so overwhelming that it pulsated throughout my entire body. I couldn't even bring my fork to my mouth without cringing. Brew lay beside me and pulled the wet wipes out of his pack. He took out one damp cloth at a time and began gently wiping the dirt off my legs. I had several scrapes, which he carefully blotted, trying hard not to cause any further irritation.

He softly tried to soothe me. "It's okay, honey. It'll be alright."

"No it won't," I sulked. "Maine is eating me."

That was the truth. Maine was chewing me up and spitting me out.

Brew started to chuckle. "Maine's not *eating* you."

More tears started to flood from my eyes. "It is, too!" I yelped. I didn't know how else to describe it. Maine had swallowed me whole and sucked the life out of my body.

After Brew wiped down my limbs, he handed me some ibuprofen and Gatorade. I shook my head at the sight of Gatorade. I had drunk so much of it over the past few days that it had caused blisters on my tongue. Brew understood what I was saying. With a simple nod, he left the tent and went into the land of the black flies to retrieve some water from the car.

But when he came back, I was already asleep.

The next morning, my alarm went off at 4:45 a.m. I didn't sit up or try to get out of my sleeping bag. Instead, I simply flexed my toes.

"Ahhh!" I cried out.

Brew turned over to look at me.

"It hurts too badly," I said. "I don't think I can hike."

Brew looked concerned. "Why don't you try to sleep some more?" he said.

I reset my alarm and woke up an hour later. Once again I tried to point my toes. But the results were the same.

I gasped in pain and quickly drew my knees up toward my chest. Then I looked at Brew and grimaced. "I can't do it."

"What do you want to do?" he asked as he reached out to rub my shoulder.

"I think we need to go to the Cabin."

The Cabin was a hiker hostel in Andover, Maine. I had stayed there on my first thru-hike, and I knew the owners, Bear and Honey. I was sure they would try to help us and let us stay there if we needed to. I never said the word "quit," but the game plan implied that it was a strong possibility.

Brew drew back his hand into his sleeping bag, his eyes barely open. "Well, let's get a little more sleep first," he suggested.

I fell back to sleep for about thirty minutes and then woke up again. Out of curiosity, I tried to flex my toes. I pointed them toward the tent wall and held them in that position. It hurt and caused my teeth to clench, but it didn't make me scream.

I unzipped the tent and crawled outside and then I slowly tried to stand. Pain was present in my shins, but I could support my weight. Gingerly, one step at a time, I began moving around. My motions were so uncertain that I looked like a toddler learning how to walk. It didn't feel good, and I doubted that I could make it through another long day of hiking, but I wasn't ready for my dream to end.

"I need to try and hike," I called to Brew. "I want to keep going."

The hardest stretch of the entire trail is Mahoosuc Notch. It is not a place where you hike with your feet; it is a boulder field stuck in a narrow canyon, and it requires climbing, crawling, and scrambling. I had to get through the hardest stretch of trail when I was in the worst pain. However, because I was forced to use my hands, core, and butt to pull my body weight over the boulders, I didn't have to put quite as much stress on my legs. And I didn't have to hike as many miles, either. Even before contracting shin splints,

I knew that the thirty-mile stretch through the Mahoosuc Range would be my lowest mileage day of the entire trip.

Warren hiked in twice that day to meet me and bring supplies. At the second stop, I was worried that I was doing irreparable damage to my body, and I was still uncertain about whether the pain in my legs was caused by shin splints or stress fractures. Based on calls that Brew made to my two college roommates, a nurse practitioner and a physical therapist, I knew that shin splints were caused by muscle tearing away from the bone, whereas a stress fracture would mean there was a literal crack in my tibia or fibula. I was convinced that I was suffering from whichever one hurt the most.

"Warren, how do you know when to stop?" I asked.

I wanted a straightforward answer, but he responded in his typical cryptic manner. "There is a difference between stopping and quitting," he said.

I felt like I was close to both. Mentally and physically, I was worn down.

A few miles past my second meeting with Warren, I heard a distressed squeaking noise near my feet. I quickly located the source. It was a frog caught in the jaws of a garter snake. I watched the snake unhinge his jaw to devour his meal, while the frog struggled to get free.

I was mesmerized by the spectacle. I had never seen a snake eating its prey in the wild. The fact that this omen would appear on the trail during my darkest hour was not lost on me. *I'd told Brew that Maine was trying to eat me!*

However, even with my fate forecasted there in front of me, I resolved to be like the frog. My journey might end, but it would not be a decision I made—it would only be because I literally could not go any farther. I would not quit. I would fight until I was fully devoured.

That night, at 8:30, I arrived in New Hampshire. Maine had finally unclenched its jaws.

7

EXPOSED

JUNE 21, 2011—JUNE 24, 2011

Making it into New Hampshire gave me hope that I could survive my shin splints and continue my pursuit of the record. I had made it out of the remote forests and unforgiving terrain in Maine, and the following state, Vermont, would be much kinder—the path much softer—than anything I had experienced so far on this hike.

I was convinced that my shin splints were caused by repeated high mileage days on rocky terrain. I had trained by stringing together thirty-, forty-, and fifty-mile days this spring, but my practice hikes had all taken place in the southeast, where the trail is composed mostly of dirt. And in Maine and New Hampshire, the trail comprises granite slabs and rock steps where the tread doesn't offer any cushion or comfort. So far, each foot strike was like being hit in the legs with a wrecking ball. But if I could just make it through New Hampshire, I knew the trail would be more forgiving.

I had to make it to Vermont. If I could do that, then my legs would begin to heal and I would feel better.

The key to getting to Vermont was good weather. I needed three days without lightning and thunderstorms to make it over these mountains. The exposed ridgelines in New Hampshire were deadly in an electrical storm, so if a front settled in, then I would not be able to continue until it lifted. The memorial crosses in the exposed alpine tundra were constant reminders that no matter how badly I wanted the record, it was not worth risking my life.

I tried to make it as far as I could on my first day in New Hampshire. The fronts of my shins were on fire during the descent into Pinkham Notch, and I traveled with my hands on the rocks, bear-crawling backward down the steep slope to ease the pain.

When I got to the Pinkham Notch Visitor Center, I knew that I needed to keep going, but the question was how far.

"You need to make it to the top of Mount Washington," said Warren.

But it was another fourteen very difficult miles to the top of Mount Washington.

"Should I take my pack with a tent and sleeping bag in case the weather turns and I can't make it?"

"It's not worth the weight," Warren said. "If the weather turns, you can stop at the Madison Springs Hut after eight miles. Otherwise, you need to make it to the top of the mountain, and you won't be able to do that with a full pack."

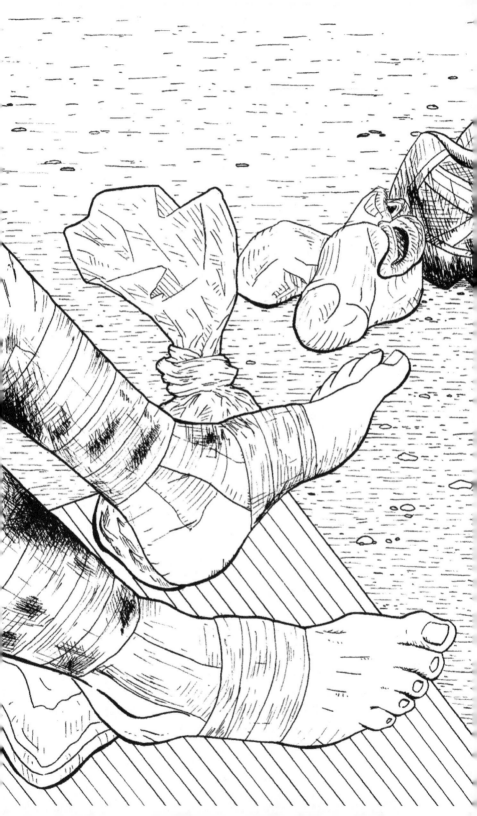

My stomach churned, partly due to the 1,000-calorie McDonald's Value Meal I had just ingested in ten minutes' time, but mainly because I did *not* have a good feeling about this. Mount Washington was notorious for bad weather. At one time, it had the fastest recorded wind speed in the world. There was the potential for a snow or ice storm during any month of the year, and there was no protection leading to the summit.

"I'm nervous about night hiking alone on Mount Washington," I protested. "And even if I do make it to the top, there is no place to camp up there!"

I was running into logistical problems because I had fallen off Warren's schedule. Not only could I not make it to a road, but there was no camping allowed around the buildings on Mount Washington, and there wasn't any camping allowed alongside the trail, either. Even if camping had been allowed, the only place to set up a tent would have been on sharp, jagged rocks. Still, an uncomfortable, illegal, half-pitched shelter still seemed better than risking my life in a storm.

"I will hike out to you," said Warren. "Brew can drive me to the summit, but he will have to leave when the building at the top closes. They don't let any cars stay in the parking lot. I will pack your food and sleeping bag and come and find you. Then after you reach the summit, we can hike down to Lake of the Clouds Hut together and sleep indoors."

Planning to stay at Lake of the Clouds was a gamble. Not only was it farther down the trail than the Mt. Washington Observatory, but there was also the chance that there might not be room for us there.

The huts in the White Mountains are very different from the wooden shelters that are located every seven or eight miles along most the Appalachian Trail. In the Whites, the accommodations are designated for paying customers, and reservations for Lake of the Clouds Hut were made months in advance. I knew there wouldn't be any spots for the two of us in a bunkroom. But hopefully we could stay in the basement that is sometimes available to thru-hikers. Usually thru-hikers will "pay" for their lodging in the aptly named "Dungeon" by providing manual labor in return for their stay. Obviously, I didn't have four hours to spare washing dishes, but I knew Warren would do my chores if he needed to.

I silently nodded at Warren. We had a plan. I still didn't feel good about it, but I couldn't spend any more time thinking it through. I had to keep hiking.

Three hours later, after eight miles of climbing, I hiked past Madison Hut. I walked quickly and quietly, hoping not to draw any attention to myself. I was afraid that some of the staff members would come out and stop me if they saw what looked like a "day hiker" heading toward the summit so late in the day. Thankfully, no adults left the building, but two young children ran around the dirt courtyard, playing games outside before the sun went down.

One of the children stopped when she saw me walking nearby and looked at me curiously. She knew that all the other grownups were sitting inside the hut, enjoying their evening coffee and tea. The sun was going down and I was going away from the safe haven. I hiked higher and farther away from the hut, and every time I looked back, I could still see the young girl watching me.

When I could no longer see the girl or the hut, the wind on top of the mountain began to grow stronger. I continued hiking, tilting my head to shield my face from the strong, cold currents that ripped over the mountain.

Every few seconds, I would have to look up to make sure I was still walking toward the next cairn. There was no defined path on top of Mount Washington. The trail was one long scree field, and the only markers were the large piles of rocks stationed every thirty yards.

The sun soon dropped below the horizon and I pulled my headlamp out of my daypack and turned it on. The trail made a ninety-degree turn and the grade increased. I was now on the spine of the northeast ridge, a ridge that seemed as old and worn as the skeleton of a brontosaurus in a natural history museum. I began to feel the clouds move past me at an increasing speed. The air felt thicker, and my headlamp highlighted the small particles of moisture in the air. It became increasingly difficult to spot the next cairn through the mist. Every time I reached a rock pile that marked the trail, I would stop and scan the horizon. I examined the landscape to try and decipher which direction the path veered. However, at each subsequent cairn, it was harder and harder to make out the route.

My headlamp was insufficient for piercing through the clouds, so I dug into my pack and pulled out my spare flashlight. I always carried a spare light in case my headlamp broke or ran out of batteries. After losing our first flashlight in our messy car, Brew had picked up an extra one at the local hardware store. It weighed nearly half a pound and seemed misplaced amid the rest of my lightweight hiking gear, but it had a light like a tractor beam. I turned it on and could immediately make out the next trail marker.

Because of the fog and the mist, I had entirely lost my perspective on how much farther I had to hike to reach the summit. I was moving very slowly over the slick, wet rocks when the flashlight in my hand began to flicker.

I remembered Brew saying that this light should last for five hours before we needed to replace the batteries, and I immediately began to calculate all the times I had used it in the past week. It suddenly occurred to me that this flashlight might be on its last hour of life, and I was still several miles from the summit.

I picked up my phone to call Warren. It went directly to his voicemail.

"Warren, where are you? Are you hiking out to meet me? It's getting really hard to make out the trail and I am worried that my flashlight might be dying. Please call me back if you get this."

Then I tried to call Brew. I wanted to know if he had any idea when Warren left the summit to walk out and meet me. My phone went straight to Brew's voicemail, as well. I knew that he would worry, so I phrased my message carefully.

"Hey, honey, it's close to 9:30 p.m. and I am about an hour past Madison Hut. It's dark and misty up here, but I'm doing okay. I should be meeting up with Warren pretty soon. Call me back and let me know if you have any idea when he started hiking. Okay, well . . . I love you."

I put the phone back in my pack. Then I stood up and resumed my slow, steady march up the mountain.

When the sun disappeared completely, so did any of my remaining confidence. Having to walk after the sun went down in Maine and New Hampshire was grueling physically and emotionally because the trail in those two states threatens hard falls and scraped knees during the day. But at night, the dangers are even more severe. I was reduced to a crawl. But at least it was a figurative crawl—for now.

My body was exhausted. Then, on the slopes of Mount Washington, one of the most perilous places on the entire trail, the wind began to gain even more strength and the mist turned into rain.

The rain masked the tears that fell from my chin to the rocks below. I was shocked and embarrassed at how much I had wept since the start of the journey. I would certainly set the record for being the biggest crybaby on an endurance hike. But for the first time in the past few days, I wasn't crying because of sheer pain. My legs still hurt, but the weight of my fear was worse.

This is why my mother hates the idea of thru-hiking. This is not safe—it's idiotic! Why? Why did I feel the need to try this record?

I thought back to my first experience on Mount Washington. It was 2005 and I was toward the end of my first A.T. thru-hike. I was in roughly the same place on a sunny, clear day, when I saw Andrew Thompson, the tall blond trail runner, bounding up the path. He had a smile on his face that suggested he was having fun. Damn it! Why did he have to make it look so easy?

No wonder his trail record had stood for the past seven years. How on earth did I ever have the gall to think I could break it?! This was no longer about the record. This was about my life. I had to make it safely off this mountain. I couldn't believe Warren had talked me out of carrying my tent and sleeping bag. Where was he?!

I kept putting one foot in front of the other, taking a break every few steps to locate the next cairn and look for Warren's flashlight beam. The fact that we had not met up made me question whether I was even on the right path. The darkness felt endless. The rocks below me were loose, and the clacking they made when I put my weight on them filled the air. I began to pray.

God, please get me off of this mountain. Please help my flashlight to last until I get to safety. I don't care if I make it to the top of the mountain. I don't care if I made a wrong turn and am headed toward a hut—just get me off this mountain!

At that moment, my headlamp flickered and dimmed. Up to this point, I had been worried about losing battery power in my flashlight, not in my headlamp! The light on my forehead did not go out completely, but its reduced power made it almost worthless. I turned it off to preserve the remaining energy. Now all I had to guide me to the summit was my flashlight with limited battery power.

I thought about Brew lying sleepless somewhere at the base of this mountain. I knew with certainty that he was worried about me and praying for me. That knowledge only made things worse. How could I do this to him?

I carried my regrets and fear up the mountain, listening to the rocks and the wind for the next hour. Then I finally heard a new sound. It was a voice calling to me through the fog—it was Warren. I kept hiking and heard the call again. Now, when I looked up, I could see his headlamp. It was stationary. I used his position like a lighthouse to guide my course. When I finally began to make out the outline of his body, I also saw the roof of the building that crowns Mount Washington. I was at the summit.

I felt an immediate sense of relief. My muscles relaxed, and my speed increased as I walked over and placed my hand on the worn wooden sign that marks the top of the mountain. Then, at the exact moment I touched the sign, my flashlight died.

I was momentarily overcome with disbelief and thanksgiving. My flashlight had lasted until the exact instant when I reached the top of the mountain. Thank you, Jesus!

But now that I was safely at the summit, in complete darkness, my amazement quickly transformed to anger. Looking around for Warren, I could no longer see his headlamp.

"Where are you?" I asked at first, but then I quickly rephrased my question before he could answer. "Where *were* you?" I demanded.

He flickered his light on and off to reveal his location. Then, in the flashing strobe of his headlamp, he put a single finger up to his pursed lips.

I was supposed to be quiet? I didn't want to be quiet. I wanted to be angry! What was Warren doing at the top of the mountain?

Now that I was safe, I was also mad. I had spent the past two hours feeling frightened and unsafe, and all of that could have been avoided if Warren had hiked out to meet me.

Obeying his command not to talk, I followed him down some rock steps leading to the basement of the building, then he opened a door that he had left propped open with a rock, and ushered me inside. I followed him into a utility closet. He shut the door and locked it.

"Good job," he whispered.

"Where were you?!" My voice was quiet but shrill.

"I didn't want to slow you down."

"But I was going at a crawl, and I was afraid my flashlight was going to die the entire time."

"Well, at one point, I saw two lights coming up the trail, and I thought maybe you had found someone else to hike with."

"They were both mine!" The idea that I would find someone on top of Mount Washington in a rainstorm at night was absurd.

"It's late and you're tired," said Warren. "I don't think it's safe to go down the wet rocks to reach Lake of the Clouds in the dark. Let's sleep here, and you can keep going when the sun comes up."

Warren had brought me some dry clothes and a package of cold rehydrated spaghetti. He had placed my sleeping mat next to a puddle of green slime that was dripping out of a nearby pipe. I changed clothes, choked down some dinner, and then lay down to try to get six hours of sleep. As I was zipping up my sleeping bag, a red light came on in the corner of the room, and then a sound like someone cranking a lawnmower echoed loudly off the walls. I don't know what it was, but it was on a timer that went off every thirty minutes. The disrupted sleep made it the worst, most uncomfortable night since we'd left Katahdin.

The next morning, I was so groggy that I felt sick. The queasiness in my stomach made it difficult to get out of my sleeping bag, eat breakfast, and pack up. And it took longer than I wanted to get ready.

At 5:50 a.m., we headed downhill in the fog and rain to Lake of the Clouds Hut. The wind was so strong that it would have carried away our words, so we didn't talk. We just hiked. A little over a mile later, we ducked into the Lake of the Clouds Hut. We were both sopping wet.

As soon as we entered, a staff member said, "Oh you must have been the hikers we heard about."

Warren froze like a deer in headlights. I knew he was worried that we would be fined or, if nothing else, reprimanded for camping at the observatory on the summit. In that moment, I didn't care about any penalty or criticism. I just wanted something warm to drink.

The young man continued. "We got a radio call late last night from a man who was really worried about his wife and her friend. Man, I'm glad to see that you two are all right. Help yourself to some coffee. It's on the house."

A free drink was a far cry from a citation. I filled my cup halfway with sugar then almost to the top with cream before finishing it off with a little bit of coffee. Warren sat down beside me. I looked at my cell phone to see if I had service, but I didn't. I wanted to call Brew as soon as possible and let him know I was okay.

"I am going to take a shorter route down the mountain," Warren said. "I have a map of the Mount Washington trails. Do you want it?"

I shook my head. "I'll be fine," I said.

"Well, take your time at the intersections. You only have a few feet of visibility, and the trail isn't very well marked."

I nodded. Then, after one more gulp of brown sugary sludge, I gathered my pack and headed toward the door.

On my descent down Mount Washington, the trail was no longer on rocks. It followed a thin dirt path. The dirt caused my shins not to hurt quite as much, and it also made route finding much easier. I followed the path down, down, down the mountain. Each time I arrived at a trail junction, I took a deep breath, examined the sign, located the next white blaze, and then went confidently in that direction.

I was making great time. When I arrived at Mizpah Hut, I pulled out my cell phone and texted Brew, letting him know I should be at the car in about two hours. Then I stayed on the path and kept hiking.

I didn't remember every twist and turn of the trail from my previous hikes, but I had a general sense of what the trail should do, and I recalled most of the major landmarks. Past Mizpah Hut,

I knew that the trail should continue descending to reach Webster Cliffs. This time around, the path kept going down, but it was taking much longer than I remembered to reach the rocky ledges. Then I came to a river crossing—I definitely didn't remember a river crossing. I forded it, praying that the falling rain had simply made a small creek swell to look like a river. But on the opposite bank, I still didn't see a white blaze. Was I off the trail? How could that happen? I didn't even pass a trail junction where I could have taken a wrong turn. Or did I?

I didn't know where I was, but I became convinced that I was no longer on the A.T. I had just traveled three miles on a steep downhill grade, and now I would have to turn around and climb back uphill to try to find the trail. In the best-case scenario, this would cost me several extra miles and a few hours of hiking. On a typical thru-hike that would be depressing, but on a record attempt it felt disastrous. The trail changes length from year to year due to reroutes. In 2005, it was 2,175 miles long. This year it was 2,181. That meant I was already going to have to hike six more miles than Andrew, and now that I had gotten lost, I might have to hike twelve more miles than he traveled. Twelve miles! That was at least four hours, and four hours was an eternity on a record hike.

My heart was racing. I felt confused, frustrated, and lost, really lost. Instead of immediately turning around and rushing uphill, I did what I always do when I get lost. I sat down, ate a snack, drank some water, and pulled out my guidebook to study where I could have gone wrong. Even though it was still pouring rain, I acted as calm and casual as a dayhiker pausing for a snack on a sunny day. This had become my tradition after one too many wrong turns on the Pacific Crest Trail in 2006. My immediate instinct was to try to fix my mistake without stopping to figure out where I was, and often, this led me farther from the right path. This intentional routine helped me to calm down, collect my thoughts, and not let one mistake lead to another. It was a Zen moment in an otherwise cataclysmic situation.

After I finished my last cracker, I took a deep breath, packed, and then stood up to begin hiking. As soon as I was vertical, the panic and adrenaline returned. I began fighting the trail, trying to climb uphill as quickly as possible and run in sections that were hardly suitable for scrambling. I was not thinking clearly; I was just conscious that I had to make up time and I had to make it to the next road crossing.

I slipped and fell several times rushing up the mountain, but in a little over an hour, I made it back to Mizpah Hut, and I found where I had made the mistake. There was a trail sign at the hut, but it was positioned in a location where only north-bound hikers could see it. I have long believed that the Appalachian Trail is better marked for people going north than it is for those going south. Usually, after one or two southbound thru-hikers makes a wrong turn, they will leave notes or stick arrows to help prevent other hikers from making the same mistake. But I was the first southbound hiker to reach the Whites, and *I* was the one making the mistakes. I paused briefly to send Brew another text. Then I placed a stick arrow on the trail, spat on the south-facing sign, and continued my chaotic run-hike down the mountain.

I was in a frenetic state. My motion wasn't fluid or efficient. I had lost the ability to think rationally, so I was not pacing myself for a thirty-five—correction, now a forty-one-mile—day. Instead, I was racing downhill recklessly. All I knew was that I had been stuck in a rain storm on Mount Washington for the past eighteen hours, I had gotten lost on a trail that I had hiked twice before, and I might have just cost myself the record. At this point, I only wanted to get to my husband and end this ungodly section.

Forcing my way downhill as quickly as possible, through puddles and slick mud, I started to fall—a lot. I wiped out on the water-saturated wooden bog logs that protect the swampy sections of the trail. I tripped over roots, usually landing on an arm or hip. At one point, my foot got stuck behind a rock and I went sailing off the side of the trail, where my head hit a tree. I thought I might pass out. For a moment, It felt like a gray tunnel was closing in on my vision, but then my normal sight returned, so I stood up, wiped off some of the mud that covered my legs, and kept careening down the mountain.

When I arrived at Webster Cliffs, I threw my body down the rocks like a Plinko chip on *The Price is Right*, with no regard to where I might land. Even in the moment, when I reached the base of the rock scramble, it struck me as a miracle that I was not seriously injured, especially since the scramble looked more like a waterfall in the unrelenting rain.

Past the cliffs, the trail became less technical, and I started to fall less often. And as the hiking improved, so did my attitude. I no longer wanted to think about getting lost in the rain or stuck on Mount Washington, and I *definitely* didn't want to cry, so instead I started singing at the top of my lungs. I don't have a good memory for songs, partly because I am tone deaf. So I repeated the same choruses over and over again until I finally reached the road at Crawford Notch.

I hiked over to the car. Melissa was in the passenger seat and there wasn't any room to sit in the back.

So I opened the passenger door and said, "Out!"

It was still pouring rain but I didn't care if Melissa had to stand outside for a few minutes and get wet. My hands were wrinkled, and my skin was pale and flaky. I needed to be inside a dry vehicle. I needed to be with my husband.

Brew had a look of bewilderment on his face.

"What happened?" he asked.

"Don't ask."

"I was really worried."

"Did you get my texts?"

"No, and Warren was supposed to call us last night, but I didn't hear from him then and I haven't heard from him today. I even radioed Lake of the Clouds looking for you! I've been worried sick."

"Well, we camped out on top of Mount Washington in a utility closet where green sludge dripped near my head and toxic fumes practically poisoned us. Also a loud crank woke us up every half hour. Then I hiked all day in the rain and got lost. I got off the trail by three miles, so it was six miles round-trip."

"Six miles?!"

"I don't want to talk about it!" I screamed. "It is all I can do right now not to cry."

Brew nodded his head. He knew me well enough to know I would not be rational until I had some dry clothes on my body and food in my stomach. I was already undressed, with a sleeping bag wrapped around me. We had been through weather like this enough times by now to have a routine. I would immediately change out of my wet, cold clothes; wrap up in a sleeping bag; eat; drink; and then put on dry clothes and keep going.

While I warmed up and started shoving food in my mouth, Brew turned on the car's CD player. He started blasting my favorite Mumford and Sons song since I'd been singing its chorus over and over on the trail. I was thankful to hear all the lyrics. I listened to them carefully, hoping to remember some of the additional stanzas for the next time I needed to sing out loud.

One line in particular resonated in my mind and refueled my heart.

"I know my call despite my faults
And despite my growing fears."

Then I joined the band and my husband on the chorus that I knew so well:

"I will hold on hope
And I won't let you choke
On the noose around your neck
And I'll find strength in pain
And I will change my ways
I'll know my name as it's called again."

The past twenty-six miles had been filled with fear and doubt. Hiking into Crawford Notch, I was worried that everything up to that point—all my dreams, all my planning and training, the grueling three-hundred and forty-five miles to get here—was all for naught. But I still felt like I was supposed to keep hiking. I still felt called to give this trail everything I had. My inhibitions would just have to be put on hold; right now I needed to keep going.

After thirty minutes, I was warm and dry, I was smiling, I had consumed about 1,300 calories, and I was still belting out songs with my husband. Then I heard a knock on the window. Melissa was still outside in the pouring rain, bedraggled and shivering. She was clearly ready to climb back inside the car.

I kissed Brew, grabbed my daypack, which he had refilled with snacks, and charged back into the storm.

There is a brief respite in New Hampshire to all the ups and downs and rocks and roots and scrambles, and that's when the trail follows an old railroad bed to Zealand Falls Hut. For the first time since entering the Hundred-Mile Wilderness on day one, I was able to hike more than three miles per hour. I made decent time beyond the hut as well, except for the fact that the trail was very poorly marked once again. I had better luck looking behind me for the northbound blazes than staring ahead for the southbound ones.

The rain eventually turned into a drizzle and then a light mist. Just before dusk, I saw two trail runners heading in my direction. They weren't wearing packs, and I was certain they were staying at a nearby hut and were just out for some evening exercise. I stepped to the side to let them pass. The second one looked at me and said, "Well, you're still smiling. That's good."

I pressed my fingers to my lips. I could hardly believe it—I really *was* smiling! I had spent the past twenty-four hours feeling scared, lost, and frustrated, not to mention cold and wet. But through it all, I was still on the trail, still moving forward, and still smiling.

I thought once again about Andrew Thompson and the grin he wore while powering up the slopes of Mount Washington. And he had been hiking in *good* weather! Despite all the hardship of the past ten days, in that moment, I felt like a contender. I felt like I belonged.

The rain returned the next morning, and as I climbed the trail toward Franconia Ridge, the temperature dropped and the wind picked up, too. I knew exactly what was coming, but the only way to get past it was to go through it.

As soon as I left tree cover, it felt like an onslaught of shotgun pellets sprayed the left side of my body. The sleet burned my cheeks. Every other inch of me was covered, but I had never fully dried out the day before so I had felt chilled and damp even before the ridge. Now, the bitter wind turned my cold, damp body to ice.

The wind was much stronger than it had been on Mount Washington, and at one point, it knocked me forward onto my knees. I was sure the fall would add another bruise to my already black-and-blue legs. But at least those battle wounds were only skin-deep. The worst pain still screamed out from the bones and muscles of my shins, and the cold weather intensified the injury.

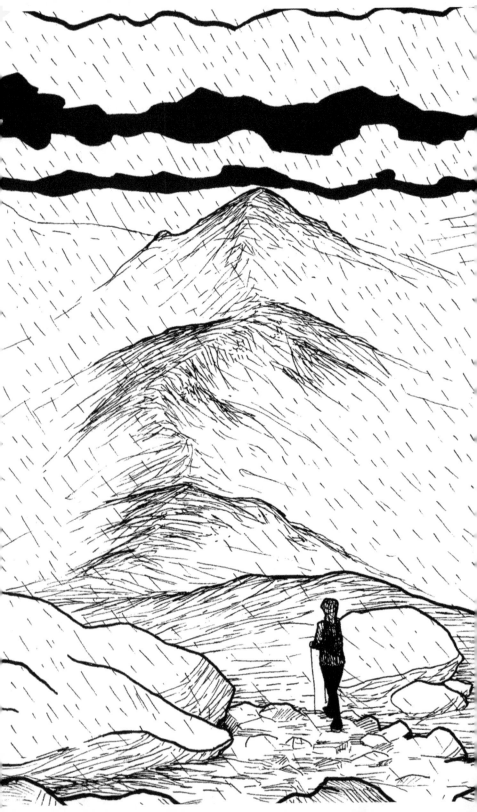

The path on top of Franconia Ridge slaloms through rock formations, and in the rare instance when I was protected from Mother Nature's fury, I would take a brief moment to collect myself before heading back into the storm. Even though I had three long-sleeved layers on my upper body, I was still freezing. When I arrived at the next boulder outcropping, I used it as a shield against the wind and opened my daypack. I didn't have any more clothing, but I took out a plastic bag that had been keeping some of my gear dry. I ripped three holes in it: one large hole for my head and two smaller ones for my arms. It was hard to make the holes, then get the bag over my head because my hands, which were placed in a pair of extra wool socks for warmth, had gone completely numb.

I was shivering violently, and when I started hiking again, I tried to sing like the day before. I wanted to do something—anything—to take my mind off the weather, the cold, and my aching legs. I tried to yell out the same Mumford and Sons chorus that helped me off Mount Washington. Not only was I off-key, but all the words coming from my lips sounded mumbled.

All I wanted to do was stop behind the next large boulder and curl into a tight ball with my knees against my chest and my head between my arms. But I couldn't. Not if I wanted to survive.

Based on my Wilderness First Responder training, I knew that I had the "umbles." My stumbling and mumbling meant that I had already passed the beginning stages of hypothermia and would now be classified as a moderate hypothermic patient. Being aware of my condition made it even worse. If my self-diagnosis was correct, I would have to do everything in my power to make sure I did not get any worse.

Once again, my thoughts were no longer about the record or completing the trail. *Just get to your husband,* I thought. *Just make it to Brew.*

I repeated my mantra out loud, "Jusss-t-t hik-k-k-ke t-t-to B-B-B-Brew."

The sound of my own voice scared me, so I went back to the self-talk in my head. But my thoughts were as rapid and misplaced as my feet had been.

Make it to Brew, get to Brew, I thought.

Then another voice filled my head. *YOU IDIOT!* it said. *What have you done now?*

I took a deep breath. *It's gonna be okay, it'll all be okay. Brew will make it better, hike to your husband, you belong . . .*

But then I was interrupted by my own self-doubt. *No, no I do not belong up here. I BELONG WITH BREW.*

It was as if I had turned into Gollum in *The Lord of the Rings.* I was acting schizophrenic. I was fighting with my thoughts to keep them positive, and I was fighting with my body to keep it moving.

Franconia Ridge seemed much longer than it had on either of my two previous hikes. On a clear day you can easily see the point along the ridge where the trail returns to the forest, but in the midst of the storm that place did not seem to exist.

I finally made it out of the wind and sleet, but the improved conditions did not help me feel any better. I felt rigid, calcified. My joints could hardly bend, and I walked like Frankenstein down the stone steps leading to Franconia Notch.

Before reaching the road crossing, I saw our tent next to the trail. Brew knew the conditions on the ridge would be tough, so he had hiked in a quarter mile with our tent, sleeping bags, dry clothes, and food.

I forced my stiff body to crumple itself into the tent, then Brew helped me take off my trash bag and the three layers of wet clothes and wrapped me in two sleeping bags. Next he placed both his hands on top of the sleeping bags and began to massage my body. There was very little conversation. I was too cold to speak, and Brew was too worried.

It took about twenty minutes for my teeth to unclench and for my arms to unclasp from around my chest. As soon as they did, I began to eat and drink. Part of why I got cold so quickly was because I was already wet. Another reason was that I was always suffering from a calorie deficit. No matter how hard I tried, I could never take in enough food to provide adequate fuel for my starving muscles.

I drank a large coffee from McDonald's that Brew had picked up earlier in the day and then shoveled two sausage biscuits down my throat. After that, I chugged a coke and started alternating between handfuls of candy and potato chips. There were nutritious foods in the tent as well, but my body was screaming for the immediate fat, calories, sugar, and caffeine of the junk food.

After another fifteen minutes, I reluctantly began to unwrap from my sleeping bag cocoon.

"Here," said Brew as he handed me a full plastic bag. "I brought you a dry set of clothes to change into."

I put on a dry sports bra, shirt, socks, and shoes, but something was missing. Brew had forgotten to pack a dry pair of shorts. I looked at him across the tent and pointed at his lower half.

He knew exactly want I wanted.

"You have got to be kidding me," he exclaimed. But even as he was protesting, he began to take off his shorts.

I pulled his wide, baggy shorts up around my waist and cinched them tight. I was now covered from head to toe. I had a beanie on my head, a long-sleeve wool shirt, and a rain jacket on my core. I wore Brew's baggy shorts past my knees, and compression socks around my calves.

"You look awesome!" said Brew.

"Yeah, right," I said.

"No, seriously!" I looked up and realized that my husband was not just saying this to make me feel better. He was giving me an unfamiliar look, one filled with admiration. "You look like some kind of badass basketball player-hiker—like, the definition of hardcore. I would be *so* intimidated to pass you on the trail right now."

Whether he meant to or not, Brew had given me the pep talk that I needed. In one hour, I had gone from thinking I might need to be rescued off a ridge to feeling "hardcore." I was excited to exit the tent and keep hiking. As I walked down the trail, I glanced back to see Brew taking down the tent in his boxers. He didn't look hardcore; but standing there folding our rain-fly in his down jacket and *The Grinch Who Stole Christmas* boxers, he did look pretty sexy.

For the first time in days, my legs felt fresh and strong as I journeyed toward Lonesome Lake, then up the steep climb to North Kinsman Mountain. My shin splints still hurt, but it was a quiet ache instead of a deafening scream. I was so happy to be dry, warm, and alive that I started to hike smart and hard. I didn't try to force my way down the trail, but I did have a lot of adrenaline left over from Franconia Ridge, and I used it all to make efficient forward progress over very difficult terrain. I had survived Mount Washington, I had survived hypothermia, and now if I could just keep going, I could make it out of the Whites by nightfall.

I reached the base of Moosilauke and the next road crossing much earlier than I expected. It was late afternoon, and if I could make it over one more mountain by nightfall, I would still be on pace to complete Maine and New Hampshire in ten days, and I would still be on pace to set the record.

When Brew saw me coming toward him, his surprise gave way to a grin. Then he shouted, "C'mon!" at the top of his lungs. I responded by slapping my thigh, then clutching my fist under my chin like Serena Williams before match point. I was so motivated that I didn't even sit down at the car; I just chugged a thirty-two-ounce chocolate protein shake and grabbed a turkey wrap like it was a baton.

If the terrain had allowed it, I would have run up the mountain. I had one more calf-burning vertical climb filled with rebar and wooden steps screwed into the granite rock face, then I would never have to experience terrain this difficult again!

The sun was setting when I arrived at the top of Moosilauke. I raised my hands and let out a primitive yell. The resulting noise surprised me. I sounded less like a cheerleader and more like a mountain woman. This time, maybe for the first time, my victory cry sounded as good in the air as it did in my head.

Pausing for a moment, I turned toward the east and could see the steep, jagged peaks behind me. They looked like a shark's mouth, with layer upon layer of pointed teeth. Then I turned back toward the west to the rolling green mountains that looked as soft and symmetrical as the arc of a rainbow. I smiled and kept walking. I was through the worst of it.

· 8 ·

THE WORST OF IT

Hanover, New Hampshire, is the gateway to the Promised Land for a southbound hiker, a portal to less difficult terrain, more road crossings, and dirt tread. The march through one of the A.T.'s most prominent towns should be a triumphant one. Most hikers loved the easy, flat road walk, but my shin splints were making me hate it.

I began my hike through the quiet streets at five a.m. With my very first step, my teeth clenched and I felt my eyes grow moist.

I did not try to hide the pain; there was no one to hide it from. The only car on the road was Warren's, and he followed slowly behind me. At one point, he turned down a side street and disappeared. Minutes later, he drove up again and offered me fresh coffee and a blueberry muffin. I took the food and kept walking.

I couldn't believe how bad I felt. Every step on the concrete sidewalk felt like knives stabbing the front of my legs. I was sniffling and gasping for air, but I didn't cry. I refused to, because things were supposed to be better now. I thought if I acted like everything was okay, then maybe it would start to feel that way.

Unfortunately, the hypothermia I'd experienced on Franconia Ridge resulted in some lasting side effects. The morning after I summited Moosilauke, I felt more depleted than I ever had in my life. I had not sweated since hiking across Franconia Ridge, and my bathroom breaks had become infrequent despite my large intake of fluids. Even as I reentered the warm summer atmosphere of the lower elevations, my skin was pale and clammy, and my entire body was bloated and swollen. My shorts felt tight, my fingers were thick, every part of my body was larger than normal, except for—as Brew pointed out—my chest.

But all that was okay because as I crossed over the bridge that spans the Connecticut River and entered Vermont, I was convinced that my multiple ailments would remain in New Hampshire.

After three miles of road walking, I said good-bye to Warren and entered the woods. I wanted my legs to recover immediately from the unforgiving cement, but instead, the pain remained and it felt more acute than usual. During my first mile inside the forest, my right leg buckled underneath me several times. The only reason I didn't fall to my knees was because my hiking poles were bearing the majority of my weight.

I had experienced this same predicament in Maine and New Hampshire. But my leg had never given out this frequently. Every ten steps, I would place my foot down and not be able to transfer my weight without my leg crumpling.

While passing three male thru-hikers at one point, my leg gave out. They asked if I was okay, and I thanked them and insisted that I'd just stepped funny. I'm sure they could never have guessed that I was trying for the trail record. I did not look very hardcore at that point.

When I exited the forest eight miles later, it was onto another one-mile road walk, and as soon as my shins felt the impact of the asphalt, I started wailing.

Brew was there waiting for me, looking on with sadness and concern.

"The car is up ahead. You can re-wrap your shins and get some more ibuprofen," he said.

"I don't want to stop. I just want to get past the road!"

"Honey, it will feel better if you take some medicine."

I had never before, on any of my hikes, resorted to taking pain medicine. I had started this hike with a natural anti-inflammatory supplement, but once the shin splints surfaced, I begged for as much of the stronger stuff as I could take. However, in this moment, the movement was more important than the medicine. I needed to keep hiking because if I stopped, I didn't know whether I would be able to keep going.

I continued to sob and hobble down the streets of the small farming village.

Brew stopped at the car, fished out the medicine, and handed it to Melissa with some fruit juice so she could chase me down before I went back into the woods.

After a while, the medicine kicked in, and the pain in my shins went from a sharp stabbing to a sore ache. I expected the painkillers to wear off in another hour or two, but after hiking twelve miles, it was still working. Best of all, I was finally hiking a consistent three-mile-per-hour pace—on dirt. I had not been able to string together four consecutive hours of hiking three miles an hour since I'd started. The trail felt like a moving sidewalk compared to the gnarly terrain in Maine and New Hampshire. This was it. This was what I had been waiting for. Things were getting better!

I left Vermont Route 12 at three p.m. I had eighteen miles to hike before I could meet Brew, Melissa, and Warren at the next road crossing. I was feeling confident, and as I hiked into the forest, I yelled back at them, "See you at nine o'clock!"

I covered ground quickly and maintained my pace for the first six miles. After hiking for two hours, I pulled out a Clif Bar and washed it down with some more fruit juice. Then I decided I would make a quick pit stop in the woods before I kept hiking.

Afterward, my stomach didn't feel settled. Fifteen minutes later, I needed to run off the trail again, and this time, it was a much longer break. When I finally made it back to the trail, I continued hiking but it felt like someone was punching me in the abdomen—hard. For the next hour and a half, I was forced into the woods every ten or fifteen minutes.

It is never fun to be sick. It isn't fun at home when you can lie on your couch and watch TV or remain stationed in your own bathroom with several back issues of *People* magazine. But it is especially not fun to be sick on the trail.

On the trail, I was alone, without any medicine and without any toilet paper. Over the next three miles, I decimated a healthy population of large striped maple leaves bordering the path. This broad, soft, three-pronged leaf is the Charmin of the A.T., but it didn't make a difference. I could have been using baby wipes and I still would have been uncomfortable. Even when I no longer had anything left in my bowels, I still had to stop frequently to let the cramping in my stomach subside.

The worst part was that, because of my constant stops and the subsequent weakness, I was now covering barely a mile an hour. I felt weak, dehydrated, and exhausted. I had my headlamp, but at this rate, I would not make it out of the woods until one or two a.m.—if I was lucky.

I pulled out my phone to call Brew—but there was no service. I knew that he would be worried sick about me when I didn't show up at nine p.m. This was going to be even worse for him than Mount Washington had been. At least on Mount Washington, we both expected adversity. But now we expected things to get better, and he would be really worried if I were five hours late to a road crossing.

This was it. *Really* it. This was the end of my hike. My body felt like it was running on empty, and after my numerous off-trail excursions, I was confident that it *was* empty. There was no way I could maintain a decent pace feeling the way I did, and making it to the road would use up all of my reserves. I would be far too depleted to wake up the next morning at 4:45 and continue hiking.

I dragged my feet along the path. The flat and downhill walking were still bearable, but every time I had to travel uphill, I felt weak and light-headed.

I didn't think I was in danger, as I'd been on Mount Washington and Franconia Ridge, because I knew that eventually I would make it to the road. I just felt depressed. All my hard work, all my dreams, all down the toilet; or rather, a dozen cat holes. It wasn't a sickness caused by food or bad water; I had experienced enough of those to know the difference. Whatever this was, it was a reaction to the stress on my body and the swelling that I'd suffered the past two days. I was going through a very violent detox.

I kept moving slowly and kept having to make frequent restroom stops. The sun was starting to set, and I was still six miles from the next road. Six miles should have seemed like nothing. When I was healthy and rested, I could easily run six miles on a trail in less than an hour. But in my current state, those six miles might as well have been on Mount Everest.

I was walking down a gently graded mountain, dreading the thought of reaching the valley and having to hike uphill again.

But when I reached the creek that divided the two ridges, there was something there that caught my attention. It was a road—sort of.

It was a thin flat dirt path that could have easily been mistaken for an ATV track, but it was just wide enough for a car to travel down, as well. I knew that I didn't have cell service because I had been staring at the empty antenna signal on my phone for the past two hours. I couldn't call Brew to meet me here, but maybe the road was close to a campground or house where I could get some help. I looked down the road to the left and right, then I followed it downstream for a few steps.

I thought that I could make out something white through the trees. I continued walking toward the light-colored mirage, then I stopped in my tracks.

It couldn't be! Could it? Eighty yards down the road, there was a white SUV. I rubbed my eyes as if I were hallucinating, but when I took my hands away, the car was still there. I didn't care who it belonged to. They were going to help me.

I started walking toward the vehicle, thinking about how I would explain my predicament without totally grossing someone out. Then, as I drew closer to the vehicle, I heard a noise. Thank God! Someone was at the car. I really *was* saved!

"Hey, Jen, is that you?!"

I froze. I didn't recognize the voice, and I second-guessed whether I had really heard my name. I *had* been light-headed, so it was possible I was delusional.

A man with a beard and a visor stepped out of the car and started walking in my direction.

"Jen, it's Adam. We met at the Mountain Masochist last fall."

I tried to imagine this man without facial hair, and he started to look familiar. I was beginning to put the pieces together in my head, but it still seemed too good to be true.

I had met a man named Adam at a trail race in Virginia last

fall, and he told me that he wanted to run the Appalachian Trail
and that his wife, Kadra was going to support him. I even remembered seeing a Facebook post in the spring that said they were on
the trail and had made it to Virginia. But this wasn't Virginia.
This was Vermont, the middle of nowhere Vermont. And to come
across someone I knew on a road that didn't exist in my guidebook was not a coincidence; it was a full-blown miracle.

"A-Adam . . . ?" I stammered. Saying his name reinforced
the fact that he might be real. And when he didn't disappear, I
continued.

"I've been sick all afternoon. I can't get cell service to call Brew,
and I don't think that I can go any farther. Can you help me?"

At that point, Kadra appeared from a campsite that they'd set
up near the car.

"Of course, we can help you," she interjected. "What do you
need?"

I didn't know where to start.

"I've had to go off the trail maybe twenty times today to use
the bathroom, and I feel incredibly dehydrated and sick—really,
really sick. But what I need more than anything is to get in touch
with Brew."

Kadra walked to the back of their SUV and opened the trunk.
Even in my desperation, I was envious of how much better organized it was than our Highlander.

"We have medicine, water, and food that you can have," she
said as she opened the labeled Rubbermaid containers. "And then
I can drive you down the road until one of us gets a cell phone
signal."

I sat down and let out a deep sigh. I still couldn't believe this
was happening. But I was too tired and sick to question it.

Kadra mixed an electrolyte drink—and handed it to me. Then
she gave me some Nutter Butters to nibble on. Adam gave me
some medicine, and because he was a doctor, it was really *good*

medicine. Then, because there were only two empty seats in the car, Adam decided to stay at the campsite, and Kadra drove me down the narrow dirt road in search of a cell signal.

Holding my phone to the windshield, I thanked Kadra over and over again for rescuing me.

"You're doing great," she said. "So many people are excited that you're out here. You just have to keep going."

"It's . . . it's just so hard," I said. "I mean, I knew that it would be hard, but this feels impossible. It hurts worse than anything I have ever done before, and the hurt hurts so bad, and it hurts all the time."

"Adam felt the same way in the beginning," she said. "I'm sure it will get better."

I smiled back at Kadra and nodded politely but with complete insincerity.

After taking one look at Adam, it was clear we were having two very different trail experiences. He was not trying to set a record. His goal was to finish in seventy days. That meant he planned on averaging thirty-one miles a day, a far cry from the forty-six I needed to cover to set the record. Plus, Adam was running, not hiking, so his days were shorter. He had plenty of time with Kadra in the evening, and he actually got to sleep until the sun came out. It sounded like a vacation.

Kadra and I traveled down the dirt road for an hour before either one of our cell phones could pick up a signal. When a bar finally appeared on my screen, I called Brew. He immediately packed up and we planned our rendezvous at the end of the un-named dirt road.

When Brew arrived, we thanked Kadra for everything and told her we would see her soon. But before we drove back to the trail, Brew took me to a state park where I could take a shower. I was already waddling around from the beginning stages of diaper rash. So much so, in fact, that I'd started to wonder whether I'd accidentally grabbed something other than striped maple on one of my many trips into the woods. This shower wasn't so much a luxury for me as it was a necessity.

At the state park, I stood under the steamy spray of hot water, shoving quarters into a metal slot and talking to Brew as he sat outside, cooking our dinner on a camp stove.

"I can't believe it," I exclaimed. "I mean, if I hadn't run into Adam and Kadra in the middle of nowhere, I would be miserable right now, and you would be worried, and I would have been forced to quit. Between this and my flashlight staying on until the moment I reached the summit of Mount Washington, I just feel like I am supposed to be out here. It's like God isn't letting me quit."

"You're doing great, honey. You just have to get some food and water in you tonight, and you can put in another good day tomorrow."

It was amazing to me how supportive and encouraging Brew had been. We definitely didn't have a perfect marriage, but since starting this hike, he had been a perfect husband. I knew the past twelve days had not been easy for him. I knew it was difficult for him to see me in pain. If it were up to him, we would be hiking twelve to fifteen miles per day, reading books, building campfires, and taking time off the trail to explore the local attractions. He had remained extremely positive, and even though we both wished that I'd gone farther the previous few days, he didn't seem discouraged.

That night at the campsite, I went to bed next to Brew while Kadra, Adam, and Melissa stayed up talking beside the fire. That was their reality, not mine. But I no longer felt jealous, just thankful. Because their reality had rescued my dream.

The next day, I woke up in the dark again and started walking. The first and second miles felt good, but then I got sick again.

I couldn't believe it had come back. I was sure after being saved by Adam and Kadra that I would feel better and be able to keep going. However, my body was still in revolt. Weakness overcame me and so did despair.

After several trips into the woods, I decided that this really *was* the end. I could not physically continue. I could make it to the next road, I thought, but I could not keep going after that. I did not *want* to keep going.

I began to question my reasons for even being on the trail in the first place.

More than anything, I believed that this was a calling and that I was honoring God by using my gifts and talents to their fullest potential. He had blessed me with a love for the trail and the ability to hike, and I felt like I was worshipping him by pouring all my strength and passion into this endeavor. But God loved me unconditionally. I knew He wouldn't love me any less if I didn't keep going. And, if anyone knew suffering, it was Jesus. He would understand if I quit.

Sometimes I wanted to do the trail for Brew, because he loved me so much and because he was sacrificing his time and energy to help me pursue my goal. But I knew that Brew would also love me regardless of my performance. And, as he reminded me in the months and weeks leading up to our adventure, this was my dream, not his. He was still waiting for the time when we could get away from friends and family, learn how to communicate better, and spend countless hours together on the beaches in Fiji. It was probably too late to plan a trip to Fiji, but we could still plan a more relaxing vacation.

For the most part, my family and friends were annoyingly underwhelmed by my trail accomplishments. All my motivation had been internal. In that moment, I wished I were trying to prove myself to somebody or something because maybe then I would have had the incentive to keep going. But regardless of whether I set the record or not, the relationships that were the most important to me would not change. The only person who I would be disappointing if I quit was myself.

Maybe I could live with disappointment. It sounded a lot less painful than hiking.

I began to daydream about what the summer would be like if I quit. Brew and I could take a few days to recover and then we could set out for Montreal or visit friends in New England. Maybe we could see Mooch, who was now a forester in the Northeast Kingdom of Vermont. There were so many fun and relaxing things we could do off the trail.

Getting sick again this morning was the last straw. I had asked my body to accept the challenge of setting the overall record, but since day five I had been spiraling downward. Every time I thought it would get better and that I might gain some momentum, it only got worse. I was asking my body to give me forty-six miles a day on one of the toughest trails in the world, and it was answering back with an emphatic "NO!"

It took me five hours to hike the eight-mile stretch to U.S. 4. On top of my frequent bathroom breaks, I also had to stop four times and sit beside the trail because I felt too weak to continue. I told myself that all I had to do was make it to one more road crossing and then I would never, ever, have to hike again.

I heard the cars traveling down U.S. 4, and I knew that I was getting close, but before I left the forest, I found Brew sitting on a fallen log beside the trail. He knew that something was wrong because of how long it had taken me to arrive. "I got sick again," I said as soon as I saw him.

Brew was silent.

I took a deep breath and a few more steps.

"We need to talk," I stated. Then I sat down beside him. Without any hint of doubt or hesitation, I continued. "My body can't do this anymore. My shins hurt and I am still sick to my stomach. I don't think we can get the record. I just want to stop."

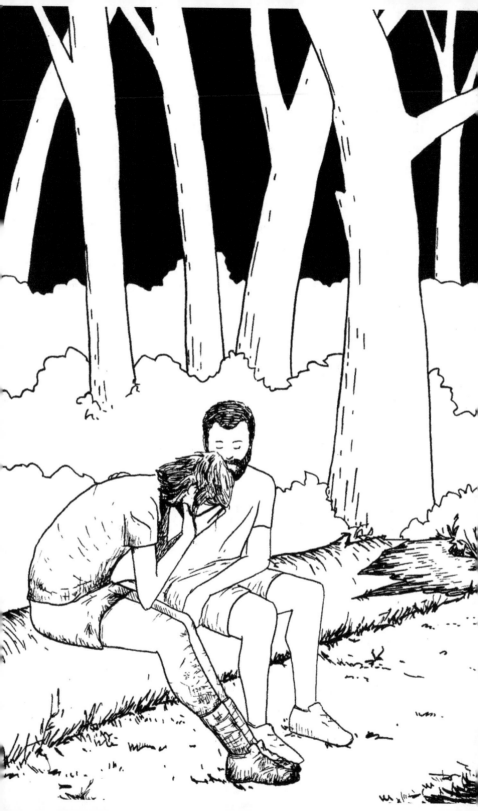

So there, I'd said it. The record was over. There had been many times on the 9,000 miles of hiking leading up to this summer that I had thought about quitting, or had wanted to quit, but this was the first time I was actually doing it—and it was surprisingly easy.

Brew looked at me for a moment. I had no doubt about what he was going to do. He was going to hold me, tell me it was okay, help me stumble down to the car and take me to get a shower and a hot meal, then lie in bed with me for hours.

I looked up with my wet, wide puppy-dog eyes, waiting for him to engulf me in his arms and carry me away from this godforsaken place. But he just looked back at me and said, "You can't quit. I'm not letting you."

WHAT?

He kept talking, but I was in utter disbelief. I honestly could not believe what my ears were hearing. My husband is the kindest, gentlest soul in the world, and he hates seeing me in pain. *HOW COULD HE NOT LET ME QUIT!*

I kept looking at his lips moving, but I still wasn't listening. I was shocked. I had created a monster!

Finally I tuned into what Brew was saying. He had been going on for a while, and he was laying out systematic points, so I could tell he had been thinking about this for some time.

"You've given too much to the trail to quit now. You owe it to yourself to keep going," he said. "And, a little bit, you owe it to me." That was good, I thought. That was almost like external motivation. I might not be able to keep hiking for myself, but I could make it a little farther for my husband.

"I still believe that you can set the record," he said. "And if you want to quit, if you *really* want to quit, that's fine. You can make that decision tomorrow, or two days from now when your stomach settles. But right now, you need to eat and take some medicine, and you need to keep hiking. You are too hungry, tired, and sick to make a decision right now. And if you make the wrong decision, you could regret it for the rest of your life."

That was it. Brew wouldn't even let me see the inside of our car. I had to keep going.

· 9 ·

POSITIVE NUMBERS

JUNE 28, 2011—JULY 1, 2011

Brew believed in me, even when I didn't believe in myself. And in Vermont, Brew gave me the harshest, bluntest, and most loving gift possible.

Twelve miles past Route 4, the medicine started to kick in. My stomach settled, I was able to eat more, and all of a sudden I no longer wanted to quit. I didn't want to stop that night, I didn't want to give up the next day, and forty-eight hours later, I couldn't imagine that I'd ever wanted to leave the trail.

I was lucky to have Brew by my side. I was also fortunate to have friends like Warren and Melissa who were willing to give up part of their summer to help me. I just wish I could have been a better friend to them. Warren left midway through Vermont, and

I was glad. Because in my mind, he embodied the negative numbers and the doubts that I was trying to suppress.

Warren knew better than anyone the difficulty of the task that lay before us. That is why he refused to celebrate or lose focus. He knew that I would need to push past the pain and emotional needs—but so did I. In a way, Warren and I were too similar.

When it comes to age, gender, and religion, Warren and I are completely different, but when it comes to the trail, he understands me better than anyone. We share a similar connection to it, and a gratitude to the wilderness for making us the individuals that we felt destined to be. He had been my logistical and philosophical trail mentor for the past eight years, and because of that we had grown very close, which was the problem. Warren knew too much about me and too much about the trail.

When I came out of the woods at Route 4 in Vermont, Warren knew that I had a miniscule chance of recovering from my shin splints and diarrhea, then hiking another 1,700 miles in record time. And I knew that he knew.

At that point, Warren and I both realized that I was going to have to average around fifty miles per day to break the record. We knew that at Route 4, I was no longer ahead of Andrew's time. I was behind. And on top of that, I felt worse than I had since starting this journey. In his mind, Warren held an image of every mountain, rock scramble, and boulder field that awaited me. He could predict the hundred-degree days in the mid-Atlantic and the lightning storms in the Smokies that would hinder my progress.

Warren doesn't mince words. He knew that the truth would be demoralizing, and he didn't want to confuse encouragement with false hope, so instead of saying anything, he was often completely silent during our time together. And to me, that just made things worse.

On his final day with us, he gave me a long, emotional hug. Then without saying anything, we parted ways.

I could never have come out of Maine and New Hampshire on record pace without Warren's help or his knowledge of the road crossings and the trail. But I never could have continued past Vermont if he had stayed. I needed encouragement, even if it was flowery and false. I needed naivety. I needed someone who couldn't describe all the long hard climbs that still loomed down the trail. I needed Melissa and Brew.

Brew offered only positive reinforcement and support. And then there was Melissa, who made Pollyanna look pessimistic. Ever since getting through the Whites, she had been hiking more and more with me. Now, on average, she was with me for ten to fifteen miles per day. Some days as she hiked in front of me, I imagined her with a skirt and pom-poms. There was no doubt in her mind that I was going to set the record. She continually pointed out how beautiful the trail was and how lucky we were to be able to hike each day. And the better I felt, the more I agreed with her.

We also identified two ways that Melissa could maximize her assistance on the trail. The first was that she could "mule" me on the stretches we hiked together. "Muling" is an ultra-running term that describes a support crew member carrying the food and supplies of someone who is running a race. Although I had barely noticed the weight of my daypack when I started the trail in Maine, five hundred miles later, those extra five pounds felt more like fifty.

Melissa also started planning her days so she would have enough energy left to hike the last section of the day with me, which meant I would have company in the dark. The rocks and technical trail in Maine and New Hampshire had shattered my confidence for walking past dusk. But when Melissa was with me, all I had to do was point my headlamp at her shoes and follow her feet.

The night after Warren left, I came into camp at 9:30 p.m. right behind Melissa. And as soon as Brew saw us, he started whooping and hollering victory cries into the night air. He handed us our freeze-dried dinners, then began his debrief.

"Great job, girls! I didn't think you two would get here before ten. You arrived thirty minutes early, which means you averaged over three and a half miles per hour."

"No more numbers," I said.

I was still recovering from the steady stream of numbers that Warren had presented at every road crossing in Maine.

"I agree, no more *negative* numbers," said Brew. "From this point on, we are only going to talk about positive numbers."

"What do you mean?" I asked.

"Well, what is your purpose for being out here?" he asked.

I hesitated. We had talked about this a lot before we started the trail. For me, the main point of coming back to the trail wasn't to set a record; it was to do my best. I wanted to know what my best was, and I believed that it was good enough to obtain the overall record.

Finally, I looked up at Brew's headlamp, which made it seem like his words were coming from the mouth of a Cyclops. "I want to do my best," I said.

"That's right. You want to do your best. And from now on, that is our focus. The only time we will mention numbers is when they are helpful and encouraging."

"Like what?" All I had heard since the beginning was how I was falling behind, so I didn't know what encouraging numbers Brew was talking about.

"I was hoping you would ask," said the Cyclops. "How many days faster than your 2008 hike do you have to travel to set the overall record?"

"Ten."

"That's right. And in 2008, after two weeks, you were just reaching Hanover. Now, you are almost in Massachusetts and you have already gained roughly three and a half days."

The corner of my mouth lifted slightly.

"There's more," said Brew. "How many miles per day did you average in 2008?"

"Thirty-eight."

"Right now, you are already averaging forty-two- miles per day, and at this point three years ago, you were only averaging thirty-four miles. To set the record, you need to average eight more miles per day than you did three years ago. And that's exactly what you're doing!"

Now both sides of my lips curled. I was out here to do my best, and so far, I had given the trail every ounce of my being. For the first time in two weeks, I was more proud of what I had accomplished than worried about what was to come.

The next day, Brew continued to use positive numbers to motivate me. I came to my first road crossing after an exhausting slog through ankle-deep mud, then I collapsed in the folding chair beside the car.

I looked at him incredulously when he immediately shoved a 1,000-plus calorie meal in my direction. I was so tired from walking that the last thing I had the energy to do was eat. But coming to a road crossing did not mean that I got to have a break. It meant that I would have ten or fifteen minutes to ingest as many calories as possible and to load up the daypack before I could continue down the trail.

I started taking large bites of a deli wrap, washing each mouthful down with gulps of chocolate milk.

"Guess how many miles Andrew Thompson did through this stretch of trail?" asked Brew.

"How many?"

"Thirty-nine. Andrew only did thirty-nine miles here. You should really be able to gain some ground here today."

Without letting my anger or frustration show, I stared straight at Brew, and after taking another swig of milk, I calmly asked, "Do you want to know why Andy only did thirty-nine miles on this stretch?"

"Why?"

Then, in a less-calm voice, I barked, "Because this section is hard as shit! Don't you think if he could have gone farther than thirty-nine miles, he would have?"

Brew looked at me and tried to appear compassionate for a moment before breaking down in laughter. I laughed too. He was used to my honesty, but my potty mouth was a new development, and it still caught us both off-guard.

Before this hike, I hadn't used bad words much. But now that I was on the trail, they had started to make sense. Ever since the first week of this hike, I had been peppering my roadside reports with cursing because I needed something far more offensive than my normal vocabulary to express how much I was suffering.

That said, I decided I might never use swear words again after the summer because I didn't want to devalue the deep, consuming pain I was experiencing right now.

I finished my wrap, chips, cookie, and chocolate milk; changed socks and shoes; doctored my shins with pre-wrap and athletic tape; and was back on the trail in sixteen and a half minutes. The break lasted a little longer than I'd wanted, but I valued the extra ninety seconds with my husband. I wouldn't see him for another sixteen miles. And past that road crossing, Melissa would help me pack in all of my overnight gear so that I could try to hike more than thirty-nine miles and gain a lead on Andrew, even though this section was, in my own words, hard as shit.

In Maine and New Hampshire, I hardly ever thought of Andrew (except for that damn perfect smile he flashed hiking up Mount Washington). In those two states, it was all about survival. But now that I was in the Green Mountains, it felt like I was racing the current record holder. We had his itinerary, and I knew where he had started and finished every day. At this point, our averages were very similar. So on a day like today, I almost felt like if I looked over my shoulder, I would see him. Occasionally, when I spotted a day hiker ahead of me, I would pretend it was Andrew and then speed up to pass him.

It was strange how someone who was never a part of our record attempt made his presence felt almost every day. Sometimes, Brew and I would try to vilify Andrew and his crew chief, JB. We talked smack, pretending that they had somehow offended us and were horrible people who ran puppy mills and meth labs. But the problem was, we knew that wasn't true. Andrew and JB had never been anything but gracious—and that made wanting to beat their time more difficult.

Brew and I had talked with Andrew and JB at several of David Horton's trail races. I always felt like there was an aura around them. They were the "cool kids." They looked cool, dressed cool, they wore cool hats cocked to the side, and they had cool girlfriends. In fact, sometimes the races weren't cool enough for them, so they made them even cooler.

Instead of simply running the fifty-plus-mile Mountain Masochist with three hundred other runners, Andrew and JB decided to start twelve hours early and run the course in the opposite direction in the dark, then compete with all the other runners as they retraced the course in the daylight!

When I was at a race with Andrew and JB, they always took time to encourage me in my trail pursuits. I usually responded the same way a thirteen-year-old would respond to Justin Bieber, with flushed cheeks and mumbled words. Brew would make fun of me, but he was equally impressed with the two of them. At one particular ultra-race, he deserted me after the first mile because he had struck up a conversation with Andrew. And I didn't see him again for another forty-nine miles. What a traitor!

There was no denying that we were both in awe of Andrew and JB. As hard as we tried, there was nothing we could find to dislike about them. In fact, if anything, the past two weeks had heightened our esteem.

It amazed me that Andrew was able to come back to the trail and try this three separate times before setting the record. After the past fourteen days, I knew that—regardless of the outcome— I would never again try for the overall record.

Moreover, I couldn't believe that JB had crewed for Andrew so successfully. Brew had taken an oath in front of God, our friends, and our families to support me in sickness and bad times, and I *still* barely convinced him to crew me. JB didn't owe Andrew anything. Yet, he remained committed to him on three separate record attempts—and there wasn't even any sex involved! Their dedication and their record was becoming more and more impressive with every step I took.

My first day in Massachusetts, I made it to a road crossing by mid-morning and was staring at Andrew's printed-out blog from his 2005 record hike when it finally clicked. I realized that Andrew Thompson's initials were literally A.T. I wasn't just competing against Andrew; I was battling fate!

I called out to my husband as he was busy refilling my water bottles. "What are we doing out here trying to beat someone whose initials are the same as the trail's?"

Without skipping a beat, he responded, "Well, honey, his initials may be A.T., but your maiden name is Pharr. So there's no reason you can't go all the way."

Good point. *I belong. I belong. I belong.* I still had to remind (and sometimes convince) myself on a daily basis that I was right where I was supposed to be.

The entire concept of a trail record appealed to so few that I wondered if it *was* fate that brought would-be record setters to the trail. I wondered if, in fact, the trail had called us by name.

Each day I was feeling more and more like I was supposed to be out here. I had never felt a stronger sense of purpose. Even though the outcome remained uncertain, I was convinced that it was my job to wake up each morning at 4:45 a.m. and hike as far and as fast as I could, allowing myself to rest only after the sun went down. And this sense of purpose gave me a newfound freedom and joy. I may not have been in control, but I trusted that I was where I belonged.

The less difficult terrain of Massachusetts and Connecticut had allowed my shin splints to continue to heal, and accruing a few forty-five- to fifty-mile days bolstered my confidence. Now that I was in New York where the road crossings were becoming more frequent, I was feeling even better.

When I came out at NY County Road 20, I sat down in our camp chair and propped my feet on the back bumper of the Highlander. Brew passed me a cannoli and chocolate milk from a bakery in nearby Pawling, and I started working on my pastry while Brew began to reorganize my pack.

"How was the last stretch?" he asked.

"Good," I mumbled with my mouth full of whipped cream and chocolate. "I passed the Dover Oak."

"Oh, yeah? I might try to walk in and see it. It's close to the road, right?"

"Super close."

"And it's worth it?" Brew asked as he wiped a chocolate sprinkle off my nose.

"Definitely."

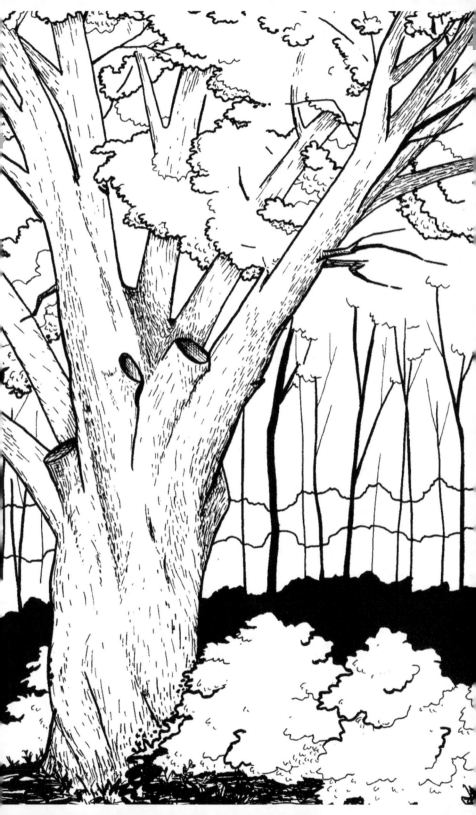

The Dover Oak is a three-hundred-year-old white oak with a twenty-foot circumference. It is a gargantuan monument of twisted branches and rough brown bark—and it is breathtaking. It doesn't look graceful, but it does look wise and kind, even more so than I remembered. I doubt the tree had changed much in the past six years, but I certainly had.

As I walked past, I brushed my fingertips across its broad trunk. My encounters with vistas, waterfalls, wildflowers, and trees like the Dover Oak were brief on this hike. I didn't have time to stop; I had to take everything in while I was in motion. But the inspiration of these natural wonders stayed with me long after I left the scene.

On this hike, I didn't just draw encouragement from the wilderness; I took my strength from it. My most consistent motivation on the trail came from spotting wildlife, tracing my fingers lightly along the surface of boulders and trees, and drinking in views like they were electrolytes for my soul. My motivation to keep hiking was rooted in the magnificent details of the Appalachian Mountains, and the more of myself I poured out—the more energy I gave to the trail—the more it gave me in return.

I wasn't even halfway through with my third thru-hike and I was already making plans to come back to the trail again and again. It would be nice to return to the Dover Oak sometime in the fall and see the wide canopy of leaves turn into a brilliant red umbrella. It would be fun to come with friends and link hands around the massive trunk (I estimated that it would take at least six people).

The strength I gained from touching the Dover Oak, and the calories from the cannoli, stayed with me for the next five miles. I blazed down the trail. The soft dirt tread and rolling terrain allowed my feet to feel as light and sure as they had on the first day of the hike.

Within a few hours, I passed Nuclear Lake, a beautiful body of water and the former site of a uranium and plutonium research facility. On the trail, there were still legends of former thru-hikers who had spotted three-eyed fish when the facility was active.

Past Canopus Lake, I unexpectedly arrived at a road crossing. Brew was not there and it seemed too early to have arrived at our next rendezvous, so I kept hiking.

But almost immediately I arrived at another road, and Brew was not there, either. I continued down the trail but soon felt lost and confused. Where was I? Was Brew waiting at a road ahead of me or behind me? I didn't have my cell phone or my bearings, and I was running low on snacks and water.

I was acutely aware that one mistake—one miscommunication or misjudgment by me *or* my crew—could ruin this record. However, strangely, I wasn't worried. I decided that if my flashlight had worked until I reached the top of Mount Washington, and if I had come across Kadra and Adam in the middle of nowhere Vermont, then God would continue to provide for me, and Brew would somehow find me. All I had to do was keep hiking.

I hiked down the path another mile or so and arrived at a stream crossing. I didn't see any signs of life, just cottage-sized boulders. However, my nose did detect something out of the ordinary. There was a slight scent of bug spray . . . with a hint of mac and cheese.

"Hello?" I called out. "Is anyone there?"

Then I heard a surprised response from behind one of those cottage-sized boulders. A few seconds later, a young couple stepped out from behind it.

"Hey, I'm trying to reach my husband. Do you all have a cell phone that I can borrow?"

A tan woman with dark hair called back, "Yeah, we just used it and it has service here. Let me get it for you."

"Do you need any food or water?" asked the man as he rummaged in their food bag for extra goodies.

I accepted some water and called Brew, who had enough

experience at this point to know that he should always accept calls from unknown numbers. It quickly became clear that he was still two roads back, waiting for me. It was also evident that he was none too happy about the mix-up, and he blamed himself—he had gotten better at cursing this summer, too.

I agreed to meet Brew at the next road. I didn't have a headlamp, but was fairly certain that I could make it there before nightfall. I thanked the couple for their help, then kept hiking.

I continued gliding down the path. When I thought back on the afternoon and calculated the miles, I realized that the entire mix-up had been my fault. It was good to appreciate nature, but I had been daydreaming and had lost track of time and miles. On this record attempt, I needed to have a one-track mind, and that track needed to be the dirt one under my feet.

· 10 ·

A CHANGE OF CREW

JULY 1, 2011—JULY 6, 2011

I like New York—the cannoli, the pizza, the bagels. And I like the trail in the Empire State. It feels almost sneaky to hike a wild and scenic trail a mere thirty miles from one of the most densely populated metropolitan areas in the United States. I mean, how can something so precious remain hidden from so many people?

However, after my first twenty-four hours in New York, nothing about the state was how I had remembered it. It was now a rainy Fourth of July weekend. The storm made the rocks and mud on the trail extremely slick, and the upcoming holiday created sound effects similar to a war zone. For three straight days, brilliant displays of fireworks filled the night sky, and the daytime assault of firecrackers scared away all of the songbirds. I continued to smell hikers and campsites hidden off the trail throughout the entire state of New York. But instead of cooked food or citronella, it seemed like every tent and shelter that I passed smelled like marijuana.

Though my experience hiking through New York was not how I remembered it, our friend New York Steve was exactly the same. He came out to help us and brought enthusiasm, encouragement, and homemade goodies from his wife Maryellen.

New York Steve is a trail-record junkie. He helped David Horton on his trail record in 1991; he helped Andrew Thompson on one of his first attempts in 2003; and in 2008, when Brew and I established the women's record, New York Steve was there to help with that, as well. He was my trail companion for part of the day, and he made sure Brew was well fed and taken care of the rest of the time.

New York Steve was fun and he was a great ultra-runner, but he was *not* a hiker or a backpacker. And Brew and I both knew he did not camp. Instead, at the end of the day, he would place his daypack inside his luxury SUV and drive back to his house, which was fifteen minutes away from Bear Mountain State Park. In 2008, he told us that his evening ritual consisted of sitting in his outdoor hot tub while sipping a strawberry daiquiri, then rinsing off in a long hot shower. After that he would enjoy a delicious meal prepared by his wife and eventually fall asleep on his Tempur-Pedic mattress.

On our last hike, after two days of hearing about how nice his house was and what a great cook his wife was, Brew and I stopped one late afternoon near Canopus Lake to visit Steve's house and test all of his amenities.

Everything was just as wonderful as he had described it. But something struck me while sitting in the hot tub, sipping a daiquiri made with fresh local strawberries. This felt too good, too easy, to be taking place on a trail record.

This time around, when New York Steve first arrived to help us, the weather was bright and sunny, and we traveled down the trail laughing and talking, reminiscing about old times and common friends.

However, the closer we got to his home near Canopus Lake and the messier the weather became, the less I saw of New York Steve and my crew. After each road crossing, he and the rest of them disappeared. I would continue hiking in the wet, foggy conditions—and Brew and Melissa would travel with New York Steve to his house to sit in his hot tub, take showers, watch TV, and drink daiquiris.

I knew that they needed and deserved this breather. Brew and Melissa had been with me for almost three weeks now. They'd suffered bug bites, sleepless nights, cramped cars, confusing roads, a hectic schedule, and one highly irrational hiker. So in a way, New York Steve was helping me by helping my crew.

But until this point, there had been a sense of solidarity. Brew and Melissa didn't rest until I rested. They didn't shower until I showered and when I was on the trail, they were either waiting for me, muling for me, or running errands for me. Now that we were in New York, the crew was taking mini-vacations, and it was driving me crazy.

I knew on this hike that I didn't have time to go to New York Steve's house. I knew that my job was to stay on the trail and hike, to listen to the pyrotechnic explosions, and to count the number of pot-filled campgrounds that I passed—but part of me really wanted to sit in a hot tub.

I could have dealt much better with my support crew's alternate reality if I didn't have to hear so much about it. Brew had the good sense to keep his mouth shut, but Melissa and Steve, the only two people who were hiking with me, did not hesitate to talk about their off-trail experiences.

It is hard to express the dichotomy of my emotions. I kept telling myself that I was happy for them. They were helping me, and I wanted them to have some type of reward. Melissa even asked my permission before accepting New York Steve's invitation to spend consecutive nights at his house. And I gave her permission—I truly wanted her to enjoy a night, or several nights, off the trail. But when she came back in the morning and gave me the full report, I also wanted to smack her across the face.

My feelings were intensified while hiking in the rain toward Bear Mountain State Park. I had traveled this section in 2008 with New York Steve, and it had been one of my best memories from the entire summer. But this time, I was hiking alone, chilled from the sweat trapped inside my rain jacket, and tripping constantly on the slick rocks that littered the trail. The sound of fireworks was now complemented by actual mock-warfare taking place near the U.S. Military Academy at West Point. And all that external noise exacerbated my internal dilemma. I was in the midst of an emotional battle, and I wasn't quite sure who was winning.

I think the reason I was so bothered by my crew's off-trail excursions was because everything was still so hard for me. My shin splints felt better, but they still hurt. And while I had not suffered any stomach problems since leaving Vermont, I still felt weak all day. I no longer had to deal with the gnarly terrain of northern New England, but I had forgotten about the constant PUDS (pointless ups and downs) of New York. Things had dramatically and measurably improved. So why did every day on the trail still seem like it was the hardest day of my life?

Then it dawned on me: this was as good as it was going to get.

There was no five-mile handicap in bad weather. I didn't have any wiggle room on days when I felt especially tired. I was going to have to maximize every *minute* between here and Georgia. As it stood now, I had to average forty-nine miles per day to break the record. I was in pain, I was tired, I was wet, I was annoyed with my crew—and this was a *good* day.

When I arrived at the Bear Mountain Bridge, I met Brew and

he walked with me across the Hudson River. Ever since over-coming the sharp knife-like sensation in my shins, I began to embrace road walks, not just for their ease, but also because they allowed me to walk with my husband.

"It's hard for me to hear Steve and Melissa talk about all the luxuries at Steve's house," I said.

"Well, you should tell them that," suggested Brew.

"How can I? Don't you think I'll sound like a diva, and a bad friend?"

"Setting a record is not about building friendships," Brew said. "You have to stay focused. And besides, if there is any time in your life when being a diva is justified, this is it."

"Well, do you feel like things have changed since Steve got here?"

"What do you mean?" asked Brew.

"It just feels like there are more distractions. I really appreciate all his help and all the food he is bringing, but last night when he brought pizza and beer, I felt like he was upset with me when I crawled in my tent and didn't sit outside and socialize. I just feel like he wants to have a good time, and he expects it to be like it was in 2008. I don't think he realizes how different it is."

"I'll talk to Steve and Melissa," said Brew.

"That's not your job," I replied.

"It's my job to make this trip less difficult for you and to allow you to focus only on hiking. So I'll take care of it."

I turned toward Brew, not to say anything, but just to admire him. I always knew that I had a great husband, but still, some-thing about him this summer seemed supernatural. Maybe he was like the Dover Oak; I could appreciate him better and take in more of his love when I was running on empty.

I continued hiking with Brew through the Bear Mountain State Park Zoo, which straddles the trail and is home to native Appalachian animals. For a hiker like me who loves wildlife, it is one of the highlights of the trail.

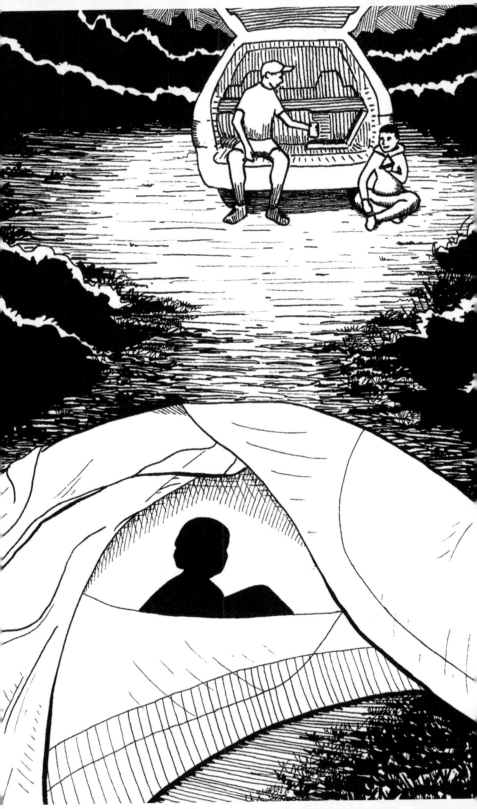

I had seen numerous wild animals since leaving Katahdin. In fact, one of the unique and unexpected benefits of trying to set the record was encountering so many. Already, I had seen more moose, porcupines, and skunks than I had on my other two Appalachian Trail hikes, and my bear tally was climbing almost daily. The long days, combined with plenty of solitude and a heightened awareness that comes from spending so much time in the wilderness, did wonders for my animal count.

The advantage of routing the trail through an actual zoo is that it provides the perfect opportunity to take all those wildlife pictures that don't naturally present themselves in the forest—and still include them in your A.T. slideshow with a clear conscience. On that particular afternoon, however, all of God's more sensible creatures were hiding in their habitats and keeping out of the rain.

The trail to the top of Bear Mountain had been rerouted and now followed stone steps that looked more like rockwork at a mansion in nearby Greenwich, Connecticut, than the primitive Appalachian Trail. When I reached the monument on top of the mountain, Melissa met me, and we began hiking in the rain over more PUDS, then across the Palisades Parkway and into Harriman State Park. The rain and fog prevented us from seeing the Manhattan skyline from Black Mountain, but I was hardly disappointed because I was enjoying my time with Melissa so much.

It was clear that she and Brew had had a talk. Even though Melissa and I both knew she would soon be spending another night at New York Steve's, she did not mention anything about the house, or the car with heated seats or the Tempur-Pedic mattress. Instead, we focused on the trail, and we evolved—temporarily, at least—from two people trying to set a record into two little kids who loved sliding on wet slabs of granite, splashing in puddles, and skiing down muddy descents. We came to the next road crossing, laughing and yelling for Brew and Steve.

Even though it was almost dark, Steve and Melissa did not leave. Instead, Steve decided he was going to night hike—for the first time ever.

Together, we put on our headlamps and headed off into the woods. We traveled as fast as we could until the sun went down, then we navigated slowly and cautiously across the rocky terrain. It was a difficult section because there was a handful of bouldering obstacles, such as the Lemon Squeezer—a narrow passage that forced you to turn sideways, suck in, and shuffle between two large rocks.

If I had not completed the trail twice before, I would have had trouble staying on the correct path. I also never would have believed that the trail disappeared over and in between the imposing boulders that surrounded us. At one point, I had to hug the base of a tree and lower my body to a ledge five feet below. I realized midway through that I had picked a bad route and needed to reposition myself because I couldn't see anything beneath me or get a foothold. I was suspended in the air with no place to go. I looked up at Steve's headlamp.

"Steve, I need you to grab my hand."

He reached out and held on to my wrist, allowing me to slide my body to the right and touch my toes to solid ground.

"Okay, I'm good now. You can let go."

When we arrived at the next road crossing, Steve was so proud of his night-hiking adventure that I could hear him providing play-by-play of the entire stretch to Melissa as they climbed into his car to drive home. That night, it didn't bother me that Steve did not spend the night on the trail. What did it matter if he went home to relax in a hot tub? He had been there when I needed a hand.

That night, Brew and I camped together in our tent a few hundred yards away from the road crossing. One of my biggest fears before the hike was that I wouldn't be able to adapt to the lack of sleep on the trail. At home, I was used to getting eight or nine hours of sleep at night, and even then I had trouble getting up in the morning. This summer I was lucky to get six, but it was surprising how well my body had adapted to the change. During the day, I usually drank one or two caffeinated drinks to help stay alert and energized—nothing scary like the small, brightly colored energy shots near the cash register at a gas station—just a coffee at breakfast or Coke with lunch.

The main drawback of getting less sleep was that my body didn't recover as quickly as it usually did. In addition to my lingering soreness and swollen feet, my scrapes, blisters, and bruises took longer to heal, too. Wounds that I had sustained in Maine were still trying to scab over. My body did not have its usual reserves set aside to repair itself.

One of the biggest threats to my hike was infection. So far, I had spent only one night in a hotel, and I could count the number of showers I had taken on a single hand. Every night before I went to bed, I either had to take a sponge bath or clean myself with wet wipes. Between that and still having to wrap my shins each morning, I was losing half an hour each day to upkeep and preventative care. And that made sleep seem even more precious.

I tried to do everything possible to maximize it. Recently I even asked Brew to "cook" my freeze-dried dinner earlier in the day. If the meal was cold or lukewarm, I figured I could ingest it faster than if it were hot and steaming.

On our last night in New York, I scarfed down a cold package of lasagna; wiped myself down with water, a bandana, and biodegradable soap; and exactly twenty-eight minutes after I stopped hiking, I pulled my sleeping bag over my head and fell asleep.

I rarely woke up in the middle of the night. There were a few instances where I had to wake up to pee, and once in Connecticut I was stirred when Brew meekly asked me to relinquish one of the two sleeping bags in our tent. But beyond a handful of exceptions, as soon as I closed my eyes, I entered another realm.

Unfortunately, my unconscious state was not always restful. I dreamed about hiking. The repetitive motion of putting one foot in front of the other continued in my head even when my body was at rest. As is often the case with a dream, it didn't make sense. I usually felt lost or rushed. A lot of times, my mind pulled images from places that I passed earlier in the day, and I would feel as if I were turned around, headed in the wrong direction. I also had frequent nightmares about sleeping through my alarm in the morning.

That last night in New York, I fell asleep and immediately started to dream that I was lost and needed to get back on track. I was falling behind schedule. I knew Brew was going to worry about me and I wasn't going to be able to set the record. I wondered where the path was and why everything was so dark. Then I heard Brew's voice.

"Honey? Honey! What are you doing?"

"I have to keep hiking . . . I have to find the *trail!*"

Then I felt Brew grab my arm and shake it, and suddenly I realized that I was on my knees, pawing at the tent like a caged animal.

"It's still night-time," Brew told me gently. "It's not time to hike. It's time to sleep."

I was thankful he explained this to me as if I were a three-year-old because I was still struggling to put the pieces together. Finally, after a few more seconds, I realized that I'd been trying to "sleep hike." Before this summer, I had never been accused of snoring, talking in my sleep, or sleepwalking—but now I was doing all three.

As soon as Brew stopped me from breaking out of the tent, I lay down and immediately fell back asleep. Then at 4:44 a.m., I woke up—as I did most mornings—exactly one minute before my alarm sounded. Thankfully, that was the only time that I remember trying to sleep hike. But after that, Brew realized that he couldn't fully rest at night, either. He was on duty even in the darkness. From then on, he interrogated me whenever I left the tent for a midnight bathroom break.

The next day, my delirium had not completely dissipated, and I was cautious to stay on the right trail, headed in the right direction. Still, almost every turn gave me a slight sense of déjà vu. That was one area where having completed the trail twice before and in different directions was actually working against me. *This wooden footbridge looks really familiar,* I would think. *Did I cross over it two hours ago or two years ago?* It was amazing how many mental images my brain had locked away from those previous hikes.

I was at a place now on my journey where I absolutely marveled at the human body and mind—how those two anatomical partners sometimes seemed like close allies, and yet, at other times seemed directly opposed to one another. I couldn't believe that my body and mind (with a little prodding from my husband) had been able to overcome all the pain, injury, and sickness that I had faced during the past few weeks. It was amazing that I could hike forty-five to fifty miles each day on just six hours of sleep. It was equally incredible that my digestive system could process 6,000 calories every day. And I didn't understand how I kept waking up one minute before my alarm sounded, especially since I was absolutely exhausted and I went to bed at a different time each night.

My first thru-hike on the Appalachian Trail had taught me to feel confident and beautiful because I realized that my body was

part of God's breathtaking creation. But on this hike, I valued
my body on an even deeper level. My physical potential seemed
almost incomprehensible—a miracle and a mystery.

One of the reasons I wanted to keep going was because I was
curious how my body would respond. Trying to discover your
maximum potential is an exhilarating experiment.

My first full day in New Jersey brought with it one of my favorite
stretches of trail. Near Vernon, New Jersey, there is a one-mile
boardwalk that spans a protected wetland where beautiful red-
winged blackbirds swoop above and below the tall, thin cattails.
On any hike, I would appreciate that the entire stretch was flat,
without a root or a rock to obstruct the path. But on a hike where
my husband was not allowed to walk with me for 99.9% of the
trail, it was even better. The boardwalk offered a twenty-minute
section where we could simply be together. And the fact that it
was wide enough to walk hand in hand was a great bonus.

Usually when Brew and I walked together, we didn't talk about
the hike or logistics. We focused on other things. Sometimes we
were just silent, and sometimes Brew sang. Okay, almost every
time we hiked together, Brew sang. I loved it. He asked for sug-
gestions and when he refused to sing Mumford and Sons for the
umpteenth time, I would usually request "Mighty Clouds of Joy."
It is a gospel song that I first heard on one of Brew's mix CDs.
It made sense that I wanted to hear something soulful. This hike
demanded every ounce of my being, and I wanted to hear a song
that reflected that.

Before this summer, when Brew and I hiked together and he
didn't have a bum knee, he would wait until we were on remote
portions of trail before he serenaded me. But since our time was
limited this trip, it didn't matter that there were dayhikers and

mothers with strollers coming down the boardwalk toward us. Brew sang at the top of his lungs anyway.

"Those old storm clouds
Are slowly drifting by.
And those old raindrops
Are fading from your eyes.

Oh, Mr. Sun, Oh, Mr. Sun,
Will shine on us again
When those mighty clouds of joy
Come rolling in."

Brew had the ability to make his voice sound low and thunderous when the song was sad and then raise it to something more upbeat when the tone was hopeful. But my favorite part of this particular song was when my husband did his best James Brown impersonation for the chorus.

"Holy Jesus, Oh, Holy Jesus,
Let your love seize us.
Let us fi-i-ind sweet peace within.
Hallelujah. Shout Hallelujah!
Happiness begins
When those mighty clouds of joy
Come rolling in."

At the conclusion of his solo, Brew received an "amen" from a man walking past us. It had been a good date. It also made me a hair more optimistic as I hiked up to the base of the next mountain under a sky that was darkening with afternoon thunderclouds.

On the morning of my second day hiking through the Garden State, I passed through High Point State Park. And before I knew it, I had arrived at the parking lot near the summit of Sunrise Mountain. I saw our car there, but Brew was nowhere to be seen and neither was Melissa. I was starving. The car was locked and I needed more food and water for the next stretch. Where were they!? They were supposed to be here. I wanted to get more supplies so I could keep hiking as fast as possible over Sunrise Mountain.

I called out, but no one answered. Then I started to cry. I knew exactly where they were. They were waiting for me on top of the mountain.

When Brew and I came to this spot on our hike in 2008, we sat and prayed on the summit together. It was a therapeutic experience that helped me to recover from the suicide I'd encountered on the mountain three years before. We remembered the young man who had ended his life on the trail, and we prayed for his family. We thanked God for the healing power of the wilderness, and we voiced our hopes that the trail would continue to encourage and restore the people who spent time there. Our short service was redemptive. But it was also planned, thought-out, and discussed.

This time, my body had arrived at this location before my mind. I was not ready for Sunrise Mountain. I did not plan to have a prayer vigil on top of the mountain, and I did not want to stop inside the pavilion that crowned the summit; I just wanted to get past it.

Out of all the images that my mind had locked away from previous thru-hikes, the scene from the top of this mountain was the one that I most desperately wanted to get rid of. But I could still recall every vivid detail from that warm morning in May, and I knew there was nothing I could ever do to make the memory recede.

I started hiking up toward the pavilion, and as I walked, tears started streaming down my face. I called again for Brew.

Soon, I heard him calling back as he hiked down the trail toward me. He saw my face and he knew right away that he'd made a mistake.

"I'm so sorry," he said.

"What are you doing up there? Why aren't you in the parking lot?!" My voice was desperate and accusatory.

"Melissa wanted to take pictures, and I thought that you would want to pray like last time."

"I don't want to pray," I whimpered.

"Do you want to go back to the car?"

"No! I can't go backward. Not now. I just want to get past it."

"Okay, hold my hand. We have food and supplies up there. We will get through the pavilion and on the other side of the summit before we stop. Okay?"

I nodded my head in agreement.

Brew guided me up the remaining ascent, through the pavilion, and down the rocks on the opposite slope before we stopped. I sat down on a slab of warm white granite; took a few gasping breaths; and began to eat, drink, and pull myself together. This was one of the only times on the entire hike that I was frustrated with Brew. I was upset with my crew for not intuiting my needs. Couldn't they understand? The demands of this journey were so great that my wounds simply could not heal.

A few miles before crossing into Pennsylvania, a reporter met us at Camp Road. I had been hesitant to allow any press to visit us on our journey because I believed that an experience and a story are two different things. An experience is personal; a story is public.

To have a good story, you need a worthwhile experience. But too many times one negatively affects the other. Either the storytelling hinders the flow of the experience or the experience is altered to create a better story (and what you wind up with is "reality" television).

I decided that I would make a concerted effort to share my story *before* the summer, and again after the hike, because it was a good story and an important one to tell. But on the trail, I knew that if we didn't focus one-hundred percent of our energy on the experience, we might not create a worthwhile ending.

Brew was able to write a basic blog about the trip and email it out every few days. But I had not held a pen, looked at a computer screen, or called anyone except my husband since we started.

I was thankful that Brew could keep some kind of journal. It was fun for him, he is a great writer, and it kept his mind occupied during those times when he would rather be hiking. It would also provide us with a way to remember the adventure once it ended. I liked to picture Brew several years down the road with a little boy or girl sitting on his lap, listening to Daddy read about Mommy's crossing the Kennebec River with Uncle Warren. The blog was more for our own PR (personal reasons), than for public relations.

I declined a dozen or so requests from reporters who wanted to visit us on the trail, and all of them had understood our desire for privacy and focus—all but one.

That writer responded by stating that it was his right to interview us and take pictures, and if he needed to hide in the woods and wait for us to pass, then he would. He made me hate the paparazzi without even being famous. I forwarded my concerns and the correspondence to his editor, and she handled the matter, saying that he would not bother us. Problem solved.

Brew and I did, however, grant two press passes based on the following criteria: first, that I knew the reporter and had worked with him or her in the past, and second, that he or she had to be a *really* good hiker.

One of the journalists who fell into this category was a photographer from the *Hendersonville Times News*, my hometown newspaper. We would see him in North Carolina—if we made it that far. The other was Keith, a freelancer from New York. He was young and fit and he loved to hike, and I had enjoyed working with him on previous articles. Even so, I made it very clear to him that any interview would take place on the trail while I hiked at least three miles per hour.

When Keith arrived at the Mohican Outdoor Center, he had his hiking shoes on and he was ready to go. We set out from the road crossing together, and he did a great job of keeping up. I loved sharing the trail with someone new. For the past three weeks, my only substantial conversations had been with Brew, Melissa, Warren, and Steve. A new person meant new conversations, new entertainment, and new energy.

Keith brought an excitement to the trail, and he asked great questions. Thinking about my responses kept my mind occupied, and before I knew it, we had crossed the Delaware River, which meant I was in Pennsylvania!

That night, Keith camped out with us. As soon as I reached our final road crossing, I dove into my tent and fell asleep, but Keith stayed up a little longer to interview Melissa and Steve.

The next morning, I kept hiking, and I didn't see Keith again. I don't want to say we made a mistake by allowing him to visit us on the trail, because I loved hiking with him and he didn't cause the slightest hiccup in our logistics. But I soon regretted his visit, nonetheless.

Keith said the editor at *The New York Times* was interested in his story. If I had been at home to hear that news, I would have done jumping jacks and cartwheels in my living room. But as I hiked over the rocks of Pennsylvania in hundred-degree heat, I didn't want to give Keith or the article a second thought. I was too focused on mileage to care about what newspaper wanted to pick up the piece or when it would be printed.

However, it *was* a big deal to everyone else. After Keith left, all

Melissa talked about was the article. She brought it up constantly, and mentioned more times than I can count how cool it was that her photos were going to be in *The New York Times*. Steve did a good job of downplaying his excitement, but I could sense how thrilled he was to be included in the newspaper that all his New York buddies would read. Brew was also excited, but I told him that I didn't want to talk about it, so we didn't.

Still, I could tell that the attention had shifted from the experience to the story. The group had lost its focus.

I didn't blame my crew for being excited. But it did leave me feeling frustrated, stressed, and angry. I wanted everything to be business as usual. We had all worked so hard and overcome so much to be in this position. I had gained a small lead on Andrew Thompson, but I knew we had to concentrate on the details of every mile and road crossing or else the record would slip through our fingers. I needed the crew to keep *all* their attention on the task at hand.

If this hike had taught me anything, it was that I needed to live in the present. If I thought about yesterday I would feel exhausted and distracted, and if I looked toward tomorrow I would become overwhelmed and demoralized. At any given time, the only thing I could do for certain was take one more step and then another and another.

On a very hot, very muggy morning, which felt even more oppressive on the rocky terrain of Pennsylvania, Melissa joined me for a few miles of hiking.

There were days when I wanted Melissa to talk to distract me; other times I wanted her to be silent. Sometimes I needed her to be happy, and on other days if she was happy, it would make me mad. I had told her before we began that I would have good days and bad days on the trail—and this was a bad day.

That morning, as she hiked behind me, she couldn't stop talking about her pictures, *The New York Times*, and how this hike would launch her photography business. The whole time, I was quiet, and Melissa interpreted my quiet as a sign that she should keep talking.

All the while, I was fuming on the inside. My relationship with Melissa and Steve had been hit or miss ever since they started spending the night at Steve's house in New York. And since we left New Jersey, I felt like both of them were helping us more on their terms than on our needs. Now, Melissa kept going on and on about *The New York Times* and referencing how *my* hike was going to help *her* business and . . . *I COULDN'T TAKE IT ANYMORE!!!*

In the midst of my anger, I wondered what percentage of my frustration was justified and what percentage was caused by fatigue and hunger. I was aware that we were in Pennsylvania, over 1,000 miles from the start, with over 1,000 miles left to go. In both of my previous thru-hikes, this state had been marked by meltdowns. And here I was again, angry, irrational, and needing more from my crew. How was I going to communicate to a friend who had volunteered to spend three weeks of her summer with us, and who we thanked with freeze-dried dinners and Clif Bars, that I wanted her to stop talking about herself and give *me* more?

I knew that what I really wanted was something Melissa couldn't provide, and that was for my husband to be hiking with me.

It wasn't Melissa's fault that Brew was injured and couldn't hike. It wasn't Brew's fault, either. It was the fault of that dumbass who intentionally fouled Brew in a recreational league basketball game, tackling him on a lay-up like it was the game-winning shot of the NBA finals—when the guy's team was already down by twenty points! *That* is who I was really mad at!

But I was also annoyed that Melissa kept talking about her photos and *The New York Times* and her career and how great it was to hike in the "summer sun" on the "interesting rocks" in Pennsylvania.

My head felt like it was about to explode. Just then, my big toe caught the top of a rock and pitched me forward onto my hands and knees. I stood up to dust off the dirt and examine what new scrapes had been added to my collection, when I heard Melissa say, "Maybe your shoes are causing you to trip. My shoes are awesome. They have great traction and are really comfortable, and . . ."

That was it. I had had it! I wasn't tripping because of my shoes. I loved my shoes. They were absolutely the best hiking shoes I had ever worn. I was tripping because I was hiking over forty-five miles every day and my body was exhausted, and sometimes it was a struggle to lift my feet as high as they needed to go.

"Mel, I want to hike by myself right now," I barked. "I'll see you at the next road!" It wasn't entirely polite, but it could have been a lot worse.

I arrived at the road crossing several minutes ahead of Melissa and in a foul mood. New York Steve was sitting in the shade, drinking ice water. It was his last full day with us, since he would be going home tomorrow. And since we were farther than two hours from his home, he had been staying at a hotel every night. But tonight I couldn't end at a road crossing, and I needed Steve's help hiking in and camping out.

"Steve, I need you to help me backpack tonight."

"No way," he said.

I guess I wasn't the only one who could be blunt.

"Are you serious, you're not going to help me?"

"I'm a runner, not a backpacker," he said. "I don't camp out."

Brew was standing over by the car, pulling fries out of a McDonald's sack. I walked over to him.

"I need to talk to you—*just you*," I said.

Brew nodded. "Grab some food. I have your pack and we can rest in the forest."

He followed me into the woods, and we each picked a rock to sit on.

"Melissa and Steve are driving me crazy," I said. "I know that I should be appreciative that they are here and that they are helping us, but neither of them will hike the next stretch because it goes over the Superfund site near Palmerton, and they both said it would be too hot and rocky. Steve isn't helping me tonight because he doesn't want to camp out. And if I hear one more comment about the freaking pictures or *The New York Times*, I am going to lose it."

"Do you want me to call Jim?" asked Brew.

"Who?" I asked.

"You know, Jim. Rambler. The hiker you met in the Bigelows. He lives in Pennsylvania and he emailed me the other day saying he could come out and help us if we needed it. It would be good to have some fresh legs. The past few days—and weeks—have been really hard on everyone. I know that you are completely exhausted, but Melissa and Steve are tired too. They are both planning to leave soon anyway, and we really need someone with us who knows the trail and can camp out with you."

"What are we going to tell them?" I asked.

"I'll handle it."

"Okay," I replied. "Call Rambler."

Brew and I seemed to be experiencing a role reversal. Off the trail, I was far more comfortable with confrontation. I wanted to solve problems, not suppress them. Brew hated conflict, and he avoided it at all costs.

But this summer, he was far more authoritative and assertive. He was showing me a whole new side of himself. I loved the old Brew, but seeing the new Brew in action was kind of a turn-on.

Too bad I was becoming less attractive on this hike, not just physically, but socially, too. I knew that the record would test my mind and body, but I did not realize how much it would test my friendships. The record prevented me from putting others before myself. And it was causing a lot of collateral damage.

That afternoon, at a road crossing outside of Palmerton, Brew and I thanked Steve and Melissa for their help, and together they drove away in Steve's SUV. It was a tense, awkward parting. I had experienced so many good times with both of them in the past, and on the record attempt we had covered countless enjoyable miles together. But that last day was a bad one, and it left a foul taste in everyone's mouth.

My two friends drove away feeling hurt and unappreciated. I felt horrible about how everything ended, especially with Melissa. She had been with us from the beginning, and her help had been invaluable. I could never have made it to Pennsylvania without her. I had thanked her countless times along the journey. I even thanked her as she was leaving—but it sounded different.

I watched Steve's car disappear, and as guilty as I felt, I knew that asking them to leave had been the right decision. We would have all agreed that the group dynamics were not working. And in order to set the record, I needed more than a strong body and a strong mind working together; I needed a strong support team working together.

I had to trust that when this was over, I could offer the heartfelt apologies, and we could have the tearful conversations that hiking forty-five miles a day did not afford. I hoped that our friendship was stronger than a few bad days on the trail.

During my first thru-hike in 2005, I had allowed myself to express and experience all my feelings openly, and I had discovered sentiments inside myself that I didn't know existed. But this journey was just the opposite. I had to suppress feelings of frustration, fear, sorrow, discontentment, and pain. At times, I even had to rein in my excitement and pride because when I lost control, I lost sight of the goal. Maintaining that constant focus made me feel and act distant, and that might have been the most difficult part of the entire endeavor.

Thank God for Brew. He was still human; he could still feel. Brew could express my sentiments to others even when I couldn't. And he felt my inner struggle and excitement, even when I didn't let it show.

At our wedding, we had included a Bible reading from Matthew 10: "Therefore a man shall leave his father and mother and hold fast to his wife, and the two shall become one flesh. So they are no longer two, but one." Until now, I always thought that verse referred to sex, and because of that it was one of Brew's favorite nighttime devotionals. However, this hike had given the passage new meaning. My husband could not physically hike, and I could not emotionally feel. But he was my heart and I was his legs, and together we were still whole.

THRU-HIKERS

Scrambling over the jagged outcroppings and wobbly rocks at Bake Oven Knob and Bear Rocks seemed much more difficult than it had been on my previous hikes. When I arrived at the Cliffs on a mid-summer evening, I could not believe that I had either forgotten or underestimated how dangerous this high, narrow ridge could be.

In all three of these sections, the rocks seemed more ubiquitous, the late-day heat seemed more oppressive, and the potential missteps seemed more perilous than they had in the past. I decided that the heightened risk must be in my head. Either my increased age or my extreme fatigue was making me more timid. I concluded that the only thing different about these sections was that more graffiti had been added to the easily accessed overlooks.

When I finally arrived at PA 309, Brew was waiting for me with a pie and two new crew members. I nodded to the scraggly-looking hikers who were standing beside Brew, thanked them for coming, and then focused on my pie. I was too hungry to engage in pleasantries; I needed food before I could focus on conversation.

When we set the women's record, often I decided to end my day early based solely on my stomach. One evening in 2008, I insisted on stopping at six o'clock even though there was another road crossing a mile away. I was ravenous, and Brew had just been to the store. He started preparing our campsite as I dug through the grocery bags. When Brew had finished setting up our tent, he returned to the car to find me surrounded by scattered and torn packages of food, as if I had been a hungry bear rummaging through a hiker's pack.

Brew just laughed. "Can you slow down enough to pass me the frosted animal cookies?" he asked.

I stared back at him with big eyes and a guilty look on my face. "You didn't!"

He searched for the family-sized bag of frosted animal cookies and held up the empty bag in amazement. Brew looked at the package for nutrition information before giving me a bewildered glance. I batted my eyelids innocently while continuing to shove cheese crackers in my mouth.

"1,800 calories? I was gone for ten minutes and you already consumed 1,800 calories?"

I just flashed a cheese-cracker grin and kept eating.

And that was in 2008! Now that my miles per day needed to hover around fifty for the overall record, trying to get enough food in my system was impossible.

I was trying to consume three times the recommended caloric intake and it still felt like I was hiking with an energy deficit.

Sometimes I did not have enough saliva to process the food I was eating, so I would have to take a bite then rinse it down with water.

Instead of delighting in the fact that I could have anything I wanted and still lose weight, I began to see eating as a chore. I could tell immediately when my body needed more food, not because of a rumble in my stomach, but because it became difficult to take another step. I was like a car; once my gas gauge was on empty, I couldn't go any farther.

That night at PA 309, I sat down in our blue camp chair, propped my scraped legs on the back of our vehicle, then with a single plastic fork, I devoured the family-sized dessert pastry that sat on my lap. My mother would have been aghast to see me eating a pie for dinner. But in my defense, it was a fruit pie.

Displaying atrocious table manners and appalling appetite was probably not the best way to greet our new crew members. But after getting down as much sugar and carbs as I possibly could, I kissed Brew, grabbed my daypack, and headed back into the woods with Rambler and Dutch.

Rambler's beard was a half-inch longer than the last time I had seen him, but he looked much cleaner than when I saw him in the Bigelows—and compared to Dutch, he also looked shorter.

Dutch was a six-foot-three-inch twenty-one-year-old from the Netherlands, and his legs seemed to start just below his neck. He had finished the trail at the same time as Rambler. I hadn't met Dutch in Maine, but Rambler said that was because he spent half of each day hiking fast and the other half reading in his tent.

Now the tall European was trying to fill the last month of his tourist visa with activities that didn't cost too much. Serendipitously, he had been staying with Rambler near Philadelphia when Brew called for help, and within hours they were both on their way to meet us. But they weren't just coming to be helpful; they were also coming because they missed the trail.

I followed Rambler and Dutch over the rocks, and after a half hour of walking, we stopped to pull out our headlights. We continued in the black night, listening to the knocking of the unstable stones under our feet.

Even though both men had full packs and I was just wearing a simple daypack, I struggled to keep up with their bright lithium beams. I kept diverting my headlight from the stones below to the hikers outpacing me up ahead. Their footwork was unbelievably nimble considering we were hiking over loose rocks in the dark.

Finally, when the rocks grew less frequent and more stable, we could relax enough to carry on a conversation.

Because I was somewhat acquainted with Rambler, I spent most of my time asking questions of Dutch. I wanted to know about his home and his family, and I wanted to know about his thru-hike.

Dutch was thoughtful and soft-spoken. My initial impression was that he was much more interesting and mature than most twenty-one-year-olds in the United States. And he was certainly more conscientious and wise than *I* had been when *I* first hiked the trail.

After responding to my surface-level questions, it was Dutch's turn to drive the conversation. The lanky European, whose height and headlamp made it possible to mistake him for a distant radio tower, decided to skip the small talk and ask me exactly what was on his mind.

"Trying to set the record—do you have fun?"

It was a simple question, but recently it had consumed me.

I answered immediately, "No. I am not having fun."

"Then why are you doing it?"

"Because it's worthwhile." Saying this clearly and confidently served as personal reminder, as well as an answer.

I continued, "I may not be having fun, but I feel a sense of joy and purpose. When things are this difficult, it causes you to change and grow. And I am learning a lot out here. Sometimes I am too tired to process it all. But even though this hike isn't easy, it is fulfilling—and increasingly rewarding. I guess, in the end, it is better than fun."

I didn't think that what I had just said made sense. After all, it was getting late and I had hiked over forty-seven miles that day. But I figured something was favorably lost in translation because Dutch accepted my answer and nodded in agreement.

That night after walking for an hour in the dark, we came to a place that was level and soft enough to set up camp. Dutch and Rambler took off their packs. Rambler reached inside his and pulled out a bag of food that Brew had given him, then he brought out a large unopened bottle of Powerade that he'd brought from home. He handed them to me with outstretched arms.

"You need to eat and drink," he told me. "Dutch and I will have your tent set up in about ten minutes."

Dutch pulled out my one-person tent from his rucksack, and with Rambler's help, he quickly set it up before pitching his own. As soon as my shelter was staked in the ground, I thanked the men for their help and crawled inside to go to bed.

But as I unzipped my flap, I noticed something was out of place.

"Hey, guys, one of you left a blow-up Thermarest in my tent."

"That's for you," said Rambler.

"But my foam pad is in here, too," I responded, a bit confused.

"I know, but I thought that you could use two mattresses on this rocky terrain," Rambler offered.

I smiled. This morning I thought I would be stuck at a roadside or camping out alone. Instead, I was sleeping on an air mattress on top of a foam pad, drinking lemon-lime Powerade that I hadn't carried. I felt like a hiker princess.

When Dutch asked me whether or not I was having fun, I had sincerely answered no. However, after he and Rambler joined us on the trail, I began to enjoy small moments of laughter and tiny glimmers of lightheartedness that almost felt, well, fun.

Developing a friendship with the two new crew members was effortless and natural. Immediately, their presence began to make the hike more enjoyable. I realized that one reason why my relationships with Warren, Melissa, and Steve had been strained was because their motivation for joining us had been rooted in friendship. They had been out there to support me, and I had not been the "me" that they liked or remembered.

But Dutch and Rambler weren't just there for me; they were also there because of their devotion to the trail. They loved to hike and they didn't have any expectations of me as a person or friend; they just wanted to join in our adventure, pass by places they remembered from their hikes, and experience the trail in a new and different way.

Both men could walk all day, and at night they expected to camp on the trail. They appreciated every ounce of food and drink that was offered to them. In brief, they were thru-hikers. And I realized that the best support I could have would come not from family or friends or runners—but from thru-hikers.

I had less in common with Dutch and Rambler than with any previous crew member, and that gave us more to talk about. We were all in different places in our lives, and we had different interests. When it came to academics, I was out of my league. Dutch and Rambler were both highly intelligent. Not just above average, or relatively smart. I'm talking genius IQs. Rambler was a retired chemical engineer, while Dutch spoke five languages and was studying to be an off-shore engineer. They were both well traveled and well read. I felt like I was hiking with two bearded, grubby mad scientists.

One of my favorite aspects of long-distance hiking is spending time with new people and learning from individuals who I wouldn't have had the opportunity to meet at home. I didn't think I would be able to experience that on a record attempt. I had my team planned out months beforehand. But Rambler and Dutch reminded me that some of the trail's best gifts are found in the strangers and surprises you encounter along the way.

I rarely hiked with both men at the same time, and I preferred it that way. I wanted a friend, not a caravan. Rambler erroneously believed that he would slow me down, so he would usually take a few provisions from the road and hike ahead, then wait for me to catch up. Once I did that, he would hike with me for a few miles, but he always prodded me to go ahead if I wanted to. I never did, though. I couldn't. Rambler was a much faster and stronger hiker than he thought he was.

When I was with him, he constantly reminded me to eat and drink. He wouldn't let me go more than an hour without taking in a small snack. And beyond bringing snacks from our car, he always carried additional options from his supply in case I wanted something different or needed more food than I thought.

By spending time with Rambler, I learned about his family and his career. We talked about his love for orienteering, but most of all, we talked about long-distance trails. All told, he had over 20,000 miles of completed long-distance trails under his belt.

Dutch, on the other hand, was newly enamored with long-distance hiking. The A.T. had been his first extended backpacking trip and now he couldn't wait to do more trails in the United States and Europe. He did not underestimate his hiking abilities like Rambler did. But he did overestimate me. He erroneously believed that I could keep pace with his tall, toned legs. As he floated down the trail at a casual pace, I had to shuffle and skip to try to keep up.

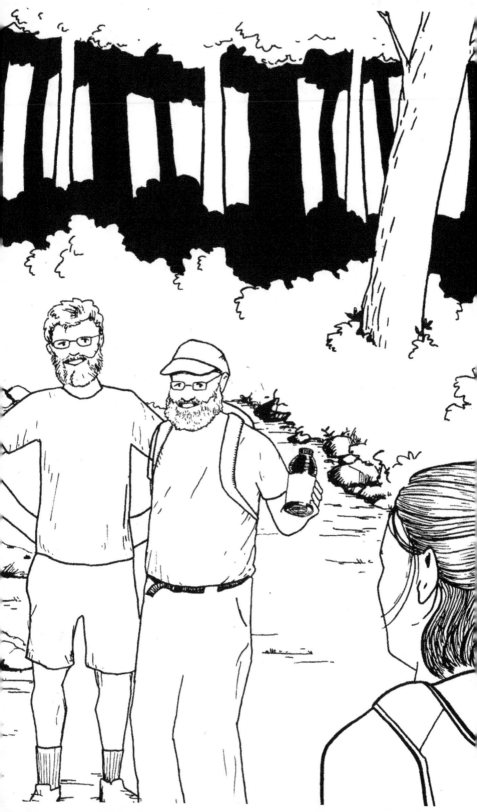

When I hiked with Dutch, we talked about his university and his girlfriend. On more than one occasion, he even indulged me with conversation about 2011's hottest topic: European royal weddings.

Dutch was always willing to hike with me at night. During his thru-hike, he often spent several daylight hours reading, then he would catch up to his trail friends in the dark. He preferred the crisp night air to the midday heat and, in my opinion, Dutch seemed to walk faster after dusk. So when daylight faded, I would simply point my headlight at the back of his feet and try to keep up until we reached our campsite.

With Dutch and Rambler there to help, our team of four moved gracefully down the trail. The interactions seemed effortless and instinctual, too. Brew was giving less instruction and was relying more on the crew, and so was I.

Often, I would crawl out of my tent at five in the morning to see Rambler standing there, asking if I needed help or wanted company on the first stretch. Rambler not only wanted to help me, but he also wanted to make sure Dutch was well rested and taken care of, too.

And Brew wanted to ensure that the lanky Dutchman was well fed. Whenever I was on the trail with Dutch, Brew took special care to double whatever he was making so that Dutch could have some. Brew loved making food for Dutch. While I always looked at my husband like he was trying to torture me with food, Dutch never stopped complimenting him on the sandwich wraps, home-made cookies, and snacks in the back of our car. Eventually, Brew started to feel like a pretty good cook, even though all he did was add water to freeze-dried meals, fold meat and cheese on bread, or pick up fast food.

When our hiking quartet crossed the halfway point, Rambler managed to find a half gallon of ice cream to commemorate our success. It is a trail tradition for hikers to try to eat an entire carton of ice cream on their own at the halfway mark. It's called the "Half Gallon Challenge." I was hungry enough to put away the whole carton, but I was too tired to stay focused on the task, so I let the boys eat most of it.

South of the halfway point, we had to face some intermittent electrical storms. I don't enjoy hiking through them, but then again, I don't know many people who do. I always told Dutch that he shouldn't hike with me in those conditions. But he always gave me the same response in his heavy Netherlands accent: "I don't mind." Those three simple words meant I had a hiking partner for some of the scariest and most challenging stretches of my record attempt.

One of my favorite memories came when I was with Dutch just south of Duncannon. We were damp and tired from hiking in the rain all afternoon. When the sun went down, we put on our head-lamps and I followed Dutch's large, agile feet. As he effortlessly sla-lomed around large pointed stones that jutted into the trail, I tried to lengthen my stride and place my feet exactly where his had been.

After night hiking for a mile over rocky terrain, the tread started to level out and transition into dirt. I had hiked the A.T. enough to know exactly where we were; we had made it to the Cumberland Valley and were officially out of the rocks.

I scurried along behind Dutch for several more minutes, then we left the forest and entered a field of tall, wet grass. In the open expanse of the farming valley there was very little artificial light, just the lightning bugs that danced above the meadow. The night sky rolled over us like an ocean. We barely needed our headlamps with the glow of hundreds of brilliant stars overhead.

We kept our eyes focused on the heavens, but then noticed what looked like two very large lightning bugs in the distance.

Then those bugs began to whoop and holler. We drew closer and discovered Brew and Rambler with our tents set up and dinner waiting for us. We had completed a fifty-plus-mile day, survived the thunderstorms, and made it out of the notorious rocks of Pennsylvania—and it was only 9:30 p.m., which meant I was going to get almost seven hours of sleep! I went to bed with sore feet, hurt shins, and scraped legs, but also with two amazing friends, one unbelievable husband, and the sense that there was nowhere else I would rather be.

With the addition of Dutch and Rambler, the two-hundred and thirty miles in Pennsylvania, thought to be one of the most tedious stretches on the A.T., quickly became a fond memory—with one notable exception.

I was hiking with Rambler late one afternoon. He was telling me about the Continental Divide Trail, which in places is more of a "choose-your-own-adventure" route than a well-marked path. I was asking about logistics and route finding and making plans for a future adventure, when I caught a quick movement out of the corner of my eye.

I had seen a lot of wildlife on this trip. I'd become so in tune with most of the animals that when I heard a noise in the woods, I could usually determine whether it was a bear, deer, turkey, moose, grouse, skunk, squirrel, or snake based on the sound that it made.

There were slight distinctions in the sounds made by animals moving farther away, but the similarity was that they almost always moved away. With the exception of dogs off-leash, mother grouses, and a rogue emu in Australia, I almost never experienced animals moving toward me. Yet in that split second, all I saw was something large and dark drawing closer from the underbrush of the forest.

Suddenly I realized it was not an animal, but a large man clothed in green and khaki. And by the time I had made that connection, he was pulling something black and shiny from behind his back and pointing it at me. My mind struggled to keep up with my instinct. Everything about his deliberate and imposing movements left me feeling sick and threatened. Then there was a bright flash.

It clicked. The man had been waiting inside this grove of trees so he could step out with his camera and take several rapid-fire shots. I could feel my stomach churn, and as I picked up my pace to pass him, I sputtered.

"You're that guy!"

"That's right," he said. "I told you I'd find you. You might not believe me, but I support what you're doing."

I was already twenty yards ahead of him, but I yelled back, "Well, you don't respect it!"

The man laughed, then he called after me, "See you down the trail!"

Then I started to cry and run. I could hardly breathe. I heard Rambler call after me, "Just drop your poles." He was taken aback and trying to make sense of things himself, but he knew that I needed to get away and that I could run faster without my hiking sticks.

When I came sprinting out of the forest, Brew knew what had happened without having to ask. Apparently the man had gone up to Dutch while Brew was running an errand and had asked him if he was waiting on me. Dutch said yes, and Brew didn't find out about the encounter until he'd returned.

"Was that the reporter? Is he back there?" asked Brew.

I nodded.

"What did he do?"

"He hid in the trees and then stepped out right as we passed. He pulled his camera out, but I didn't know if it was a camera or a gun or what! I have never felt so, so . . ."

I was struggling to find the words that summed up the sick feeling in my stomach. The hair on my arms was standing on end, my heart was beating out of my chest, and I had an overwhelming sense of danger.

"Violated?" Brew suggested.

"Yes, violated," I said.

We heard a noise and turned. It was Rambler coming out of the woods with my hiking sticks. I knew I needed to get going because the photographer wouldn't be far behind.

"I need to leave. I need to go *right now*," I said.

"You need to sit down and eat something," said Brew.

"I can't. I don't want to see him again."

I started crying again as Brew handed me a McDonald's chicken sandwich and a drink from the car.

"Alright, go. I'll take care of this, and I'll meet you at the next road crossing."

I sped off into the woods. It was one of the only times on the entire hike that I bypassed a rest stop, and it was also one of the only times that I ran.

When my pace and my heart rate began to slow down, I tried to rationalize what had just happened. Maybe it wasn't so bad. It was just a reporter trying to take a few pictures of me on a public hiking trail. What was so hostile about that?

But my attempts to justify what had happened did not work. Ever since my first correspondence with this particular journalist, he had acted aggressively and had ignored any requests I made or boundaries I put in place. His editor told me that she had handled the situation and asked him not to come to the trail to take any pictures. But obviously, he had disregarded her wishes as well. We had not been giving live updates on our location, so that meant this stranger had been doing some pretty heavy recon to pinpoint our whereabouts—and the fact that he had hidden in the forest and jumped out at us right when we passed made me furious.

In my backpacking clinics, I always told women that one key to staying safe on the trail is to trust your instincts. And my instincts, my intuition, every ounce of my being were screaming at me to stay as far away from this man as possible. But how could I make sure that he stayed away from me?

Two hours passed. I helped a confused backpacker with directions, and I also spotted a black bear. I felt safe deep within the forest. I knew based on this guy's oversized stomach that he would only be a threat near the road crossings. But as the sun started to hang low in the sky and every step brought me closer to PA 501, my anxiety returned. Then I heard a noise up ahead. I looked down the trail and saw a lean hiker taking long, quick strides in my direction.

"Dutch!"

I was relieved to see my new friend, and I quickly rushed to his side. I wanted to hug him and thank him for coming in to find me, but both Dutch and Rambler were shy when it came to receiving praise or affection, so I settled for hiking on his heels.

"How are you doing?" Dutch inquired.

"I am pissed—and a little scared. . . ." My first few words sounded mean, and my final word sounded shaky. I stopped to take a deep breath. "Thanks for hiking in to meet me." My voice remained wobbly, but I continued. "Did the photographer come out of the woods when I left?"

"Yeah. He tried to hide just inside the forest for a little bit, but Brew saw him."

"Then what happened?" I no longer stuttered. And, now, it was Dutch who paused and took a deep breath. "Dutch! What happened next?"

"Well, Brew and the reporter got into an argument. Brew asked him to leave you alone, and he said no. Then Brew threatened to call the police. At that point the photographer started screaming and cursing at Brew. He was very angry."

"What did you and Rambler do?"

"We stood at the car and watched."

Dutch's honest, straightforward answers helped me set the scene. I could clearly picture my two brilliant, pacifist thru-hiker friends standing awkwardly behind the protection of an open car door, glancing at each other with wide eyes. The thing was, normally Brew would have been standing there with them. For as long as I'd known him, I had never once heard him raise his voice to another person. He only yelled after the Tar Heels lost important basketball games, and even then, he directed it at the TV.

"Well, how did it end?"

"Brew wrote down the man's license-plate number and then called the police. The photographer got in his car and continued screaming at Brew as he drove away."

Now that I felt safe with Dutch and knew that my husband had stood up for me, I immediately went from feeling scared to feeling strangely excited.

I was shocked and a little surprised at how confident and authoritative my husband had been during the incident. He had just defended my honor. He had protected me. Once again, this was a side of him I had never seen before—and I liked it!

When we met Brew and Rambler at the road, I ran into Brew's arms. I don't know if his lean, wiry frame had ever felt so safe or comforting.

With my head tucked beneath his chin, my husband filled me in on the remaining details in his usual soft tone.

"Everything is going to be all right. I called the local police and filed a report. I gave them the photographer's name and license-plate number and they were going to try to find him and warn him that if he continued to follow us down the trail, we could file harassment charges."

I lifted my head and looked my husband in the eyes. "So you really raised your voice at him?" I asked.

"I was stern," Brew demurred.

"And he basically cussed you out?"

"Yeah," Brew chuckled. "All while grandstanding about professional integrity and how I should respect his right to take pictures."

"But you never cursed at him?"

"No," said Brew. "If teaching five years of inner-city middle school prepared me for one moment on this hike, then that was it."

"Do you think he'll bother us anymore?"

"He better not," Brew responded.

I squeezed my husband's neck even tighter. I could never do this without him. Then, for only the second time since we started the hike, we got a hotel room.

When we reached the Mason-Dixon Line, my aunt and uncle greeted us at Pen-Mar State Park. As soon as my aunt spotted me, she ran down the trail with her arms wide open. My mom's older sister had always been supportive of my hiking endeavors. For the past eight years, she had encouraged me by providing food for the trail and what she called "food for thought," which consisted of newspaper clippings and magazine articles that I could read in my tent at night.

That afternoon, after embracing me and all the sweat and stench that covered my body, she led me over to my uncle, who was stationed next to a blanket in the shade. On the blanket was a buffet of berries, tortilla chips, and guacamole. My aunt had gone out on a limb and even purchased a container of gluten-free brownies from a local health food co-op. Being able to enjoy a brief family picnic near the halfway point of this grueling journey was the best gift I could have received. I don't think anything would have lifted my spirits in quite the same way. But sitting there in the shade on that soft blanket, shoving handfuls of blueberries into my mouth, I began to miss my mom.

I used to really struggle with the fact that my mom did not support my love of backpacking. But as I grew older, I began to understand it more.

Over the years, she has become more accustomed to the trail. She no longer thinks that it is *as* dangerous or unsafe as she did when I first started backpacking. And Brew's companionship on my journeys provides her with more peace of mind. I think after eight years, she's even beginning to understand why I want, or need, to be in the woods. But she still feels helpless.

My mom knows that the trail is going to be hard on me. She knows that I am going to hurt, and, worst of all, she knows that there is nothing she can do about it. My mom does not like feeling weak. Like a mama bear, she is stubborn, territorial, and protective. And as Brew likes to remind me, the apple doesn't fall far from the tree.

Entering the south marked the third and final phase of our journey.

Phase one focused on survival. The first twelve days, hiking from Maine to Vermont, had been about enduring the most difficult terrain and conditions on the entire trail.

During phase two, the goal was to gain a lead. Every day between Vermont and Pennsylvania, our intention was to travel a little farther than Andrew Thompson had in 2005. Some days, I would hike a few miles farther, other days I just stumbled a few steps past where he'd slept. Our strategy and our persistence had worked. Now that we were in the southeast, we had gained almost a full day on Andrew's record.

In Maryland we started our last and longest phase. For the next three weeks, our objective would be to hold steady and maintain our lead—something that would be easier said than done.

Maintaining our position from this point forward would be more difficult than it had been to gain an advantage. I was completely worn down, and I was well aware of the fact that Andrew lit through the South like Sherman's army. On a positive note, the Mason-Dixon Line marked the first time since we'd been in Maine that I was not feeling my shin splints on a daily basis. My legs had been on the mend since reaching Vermont, but it took over 1,200 miles before I could stop taping them altogether. For the past six states, I worried daily that the slightest tweak or misstep could send me back into a state of misery.

From the beginning, my strategy had been to *hike* the majority of my miles. However, I had always believed that when I reached milder terrain in the mid-Atlantic and southern section, I would need to run short sections in order to compete with the trail runners who had set records in the past.

Now, even though my shin splints were healed, I had lost the ability and desire to run. My running muscles had realigned themselves to support my hiking motion. And, more importantly, my thoughts had shifted, too. It was clear to me now that I did not *need* to run to set the record.

Looking back, it seemed that the shins splints were a sadistic blessing. The pain taught me to pace myself and kept me from running on the first half of the hike, and this reduced the risk of injuries or falls. It also made me rely on my hiking poles, which protected my joints from some of the pounding I asked my body to endure each day. In Maryland, I no longer believed that an inability to run was a disadvantage; if anything, my odds of setting the record *increased* once I realized that I could accomplish my goal just by hiking.

It was hard for our friends and critics to believe that we could cover our daily mileage without even an occasional jog. But beyond trying to escape the unwanted reporter in Pennsylvania, my gait never increased. A writer for *Runner's World* magazine kept calling and asking Brew how much I was running, and Brew had to keep telling him, "She's not." The reporter refused to believe him and pressed him for a percentage of miles that I was running each day.

Sometimes Brew would joke with me as I neared the car, "C'mon! Here we go. Five strides. You can do it! If you run you can have an article in *Runner's World*. I'll call the reporter and tell him right now that my wife just ran 0.001% of the Appalachian Trail."

I couldn't help but laugh when Brew implored me to run. Then I would look at his smiling face and meet his knowing, confident gaze. Together we had taken ownership of this hike. We were no longer following someone else's footsteps. Brew was secure in his role as the crew chief, and I had proved to myself that I could set the record. We weren't operating the same way that Warren or Horton or Andrew had when they set the record. The men who had been my trail heroes and mentors were becoming my peers.

Our routine also did not involve following the precise schedule that Warren had left for us. Instead, we set daily goals each morning, but we always remained flexible. I would put in long, efficient, consistent days. And Brew would meet me as much as possible, help me focus on positive numbers, and solicit extra help along the way—lots of extra help. If one thing differentiated my hike from previous records, it was that we were receiving far more support.

There are many traditional aspects of backpacking that you don't experience on a record attempt. But one thing that seemed consistent was sharing intimate moments and building close friendships.

I depended on, appreciated, and cared for the people who I shared the trail with more on this hike than on any other. If Brew had not torn his ACL, we would not have asked for additional help, and we probably would not have been ahead of Andrew Thompson. Brew's injury, like mine, now seemed to be a blessing in disguise.

I needed old friends like Warren, Melissa, and New York Steve to make it through the difficult transition at the start of the trail. Dutch and Rambler reaffirmed the idea that offering support could be enjoyable for both parties. They also helped us survive the mid-Atlantic. Unfortunately, Brew and I knew that Rambler would be leaving us soon, and that Dutch would follow him within the week. I hated to see them go, but their impending departure coincided with the arrival of one of my favorite people.

From the moment we left Katahdin, I had been eagerly anticipating the arrival of David Horton.

Sharing the trail with David Horton is always a memorable experience, so I was elated when he arrived to help us.

He appeared on the heels of completing a 3,000-mile bike race along the Continental Divide Trail and was still worn-out from his adventure and nursing a bum knee. I knew that he was exhausted and hurt, but I didn't think it would matter. I still had Rambler and Dutch hiking with me for a few more days so I didn't need Horton nearly as much on the trail as at the road crossings. Horton was one of the best and most enthusiastic motivators that I had ever known. And I needed all the encouragement that I could get.

However, even Horton's encouragement couldn't change the high temperatures. Since we had reached Maryland, every moment of every day had been unbearably hot. The highs were in the upper nineties. I started pouring sweat the moment I stepped out of my tent and didn't stop until fifteen or sixteen hours later. My skin glistened with water and white salt crystals. For the first time in my life, I took sodium pills to try to keep my electrolytes balanced. But I still felt depleted. I also felt nauseous—really nauseous.

On our second day in Virginia, I encountered the "Roller-coaster," a thirteen-mile stretch of trail with six steep climbs and six sudden descents. There was no level terrain in the Rollercoaster and no place to rest. Dutch and I hiked through this section during the hottest part of the day. It was the only time I hiked with him when I felt like the stronger half. The temperature was oppressive to me, and I had grown up in the South. For Dutch, coming from the mild climate of Northern Europe, the hot, heavy air was unbearable. It felt as if we were choking on it instead of breathing it. Toward the end of every climb, Dutch had to stop and bend over with his hands on his knees while I continued to stumble down the trail feeling as if I was going to throw up.

When we exited the Rollercoaster and reached the next road crossing, Dutch and I both collapsed.

Dutch turned to Brew and said, "Do you have any ice in the car that I could have?" It was the first time since joining us in Pennsylvania that Dutch had actually asked for something.

Brew dug into the cooler and handed a clear, frozen chunk to Dutch, who then held the dripping slab on the back of his neck as it melted.

In the meantime, I had taken off my shirt and was sitting in our camp chair in my sports bra and shorts. Rambler held a news-paper over my head to try and provide some shade.

Brew came over to me, put his hand on my shoulder, and asked, "Do you need anything?"

"Don't touch!" I gasped, and he quickly removed his hand.

It was still too hot for affection. Even my husband's gentle fin-gers seemed to burn my skin.

"I don't think I have ever seen you struggle so much with heat," said Horton.

"That's because I've never felt heat like *this* before," I replied.

I thought I knew heat, but that day in northern Virginia seemed to redefine the word. It was much worse than anything

I had experienced in the desert of Southern California or in Australia's bush country. It felt like I was competing in the Badwater Ultramarathon through Death Valley. Except that I knew after I finished this race, I would have to wake up and run it again tomorrow.

That night in our tent, I slept naked without my sleeping bag in an effort to stay cool. Brew was extremely receptive to my cooling technique, but unfortunately for him, not even the darkness brought relief. It was still too hot to touch.

The next morning I woke up, drank a protein drink and continued down the trail. The vanilla Ensure that I consumed at the tent seemed stuck between my throat and my chest. I wanted it to go down, but it wanted to come back up.

I took some deep breaths in an attempt to force the shake into my stomach, but it didn't work. The upchuck was imminent, and tears were welling up in the corner of my eyes.

"Keep it down," I whispered. "Keep it down."

I needed those calories and I hated—I mean *hated*—throwing up. Even when I was violently ill in Vermont, I told myself that at least it was diarrhea and not vomit. At home, my efforts to avoid puking always led me to cut off any food intake once nausea set in, but out here I *had* to keep eating.

Thankfully Horton was used to helping exhausted ultra-runners through such illnesses. At the next road he replaced my Clif Bar and fruit juice with doughnut holes and Powerade, and miraculously, the sugary snacks provided almost instant relief. Talk about alternative medicine!

When I stood up, I felt good enough to give Rambler a hug and say good-bye without worrying about leaving a present on his shirt. Brew and I thanked him profusely as he blushed and rushed over to his car to end the praise. Then our short, scraggly thru-hiker friend left, just as quickly and unpretentiously as he had arrived.

I wished Rambler didn't have to leave, but I felt certain that I would hike with him again. Brew and I both agreed that Rambler had been the crew's MVH, or Most Valuable Hiker. He had come to the trail when we desperately needed help, he was always willing to hike—even at 4:45 a.m.—*and* he had brought Dutch. He also left Dutch, who was able to stay an additional three days. I planned to make the most of his remaining time with us. And together we entered into Shenandoah National Park.

Dutch and I started our stretch in silence, but as the doughnut holes and Powerade started to wear off, I immediately struck up a conversation to take my mind off my returning nausea.

"Dutch, what are you thinking about right now?" I demanded.

In his subtle voice, he responded, "Oh, I was just thinking about what I would do differently if I were the one trying to set the record."

I laughed. This conversation was *definitely* going to take my mind off of my stomach.

"So, what would you do differently?" I inquired.

"Well, you like to eat protein in the morning. I would eat more carbohydrates like oatmeal and rice, and I would eat pasta during the day."

"What about doughnut holes and Gatorade?"

"Ha. Yes, maybe if I were sick."

"What else? Tell me more!"

"Well," he said, "I think I would hike like you, not run. And I would want my girlfriend here to take care of me, like Brew is taking care of you. But she couldn't do all the planning and logistics that Brew does, so I would need other friends to help with that. Maybe you could help with that?"

"I'm in," I replied. "So would you ever do it?"

"Maybe on a shorter trail," he said. "I don't know that I would want to try for a record on something as long as this."

Although it seemed unlikely that my friend from the Netherlands would ever come back to the states and try for an A.T. record, in my mind, I couldn't handpick a better candidate. And I meant what I had said; I would be the first to volunteer for his crew.

After giving so much to this record attempt, it made me realize that I *did* have a preference for who I would like to go after record attempts in the future.

HYOH is a common acronym on the trail. It stands for "Hike Your Own Hike," and it is one of the most insincere statements that I've ever heard. Hikers use it the same way Southerners say "bless her heart." It is just a gentle tagline at the end of an insult.

When I heard the phrase "hike your own hike," it was usually preceded by one of the following statements: "You should never hike with a dog," "females shouldn't hike alone," "no one should carry more than thirty pounds in their pack," "people with less than twenty pounds in their pack are crazy," and my current favorite, "I don't agree with record attempts."

I respected hikers who owned their opinions far more than those who finished their critique of my hike with a fake peace offering.

Forget HYOH. I now had a clear vision of the type of person I wanted to attempt records in the future. Ideally, it would be someone who had completed the A.T. *before* trying to set a record on it. I would also want someone like Dutch, who was extremely humble. He or she needed to respect the people who set records in the past. But most of all, I just wanted it to be someone who really loved the Appalachian Trail. I would hate it if the record was just something for someone to check off a list.

I was going after the record in a very different manner than Andrew did in 2005. I wasn't running nearly as much as Horton had when he set the mark in 1991, and I certainly wasn't as numbers-focused as Warren had been when he established the record in the seventies. But I knew these three record holders, and I knew that they loved the trail. They were devoted to it before their record attempts, and they kept a relationship with it after they finished.

Warren had hiked the trail over sixteen times and was actively working on number seventeen. Horton had done trail maintenance on the A.T. for over twenty years, and Andrew moved to a house in New Hampshire that backed up to the White Mountains. Critics who mistakenly believe that a record holder cannot really appreciate their time or experience on the trail have obviously never crossed paths with these men.

Another personality trait that stood out about these three previous record holders was that they had all been supportive of my endeavor. Warren had agreed to help us for twelve days at the start of our journey, and he wanted me to succeed so badly that when I was injured and sick, I felt like I was letting him down.

Andrew, on the other hand, had clearly stated that he did not want me to break his record. But at the same time, he had provided us with his daily mileage and blog, offered to come and hike with us in New Hampshire (even though he was out of town when we passed through), and called Brew three or four times to check on our progress. Sure, he wasn't sitting at home cheering me on, but he wasn't standing in my way, either.

Then there was Horton. No one was more vocal about his love of the A.T.—in fact, no one was more vocal, period—than David Horton. That is why it was somewhat surprising to come to the next road crossing and find him so subdued.

"Hey, Horty, whatcha up to?" I asked.

"Not much," he replied. "I got some more doughnut holes here if you want some."

"Thanks!" I took the doughnut holes, offered some to Dutch, then began popping them in my mouth one by one.

"I'm going to take a break for the next few hours," Horton informed me. "Brew went to get some groceries and do laundry, but he'll meet you at the next few road crossings. And you have Dutch with you, so you'll be fine."

I looked at Dutch and winked. "Yep, me and long-legs over here. We'll be fine unless he hikes me into the ground."

"Well, you should try to run a little, then maybe you could keep up," suggested Horton.

"Uh-uh," I said with my mouth full of glazed pastries. "Don't need to run. Don't want to run."

"Well, you are lucky to have so much help," Horton continued. "I never had anyone like Dutch helping me and carrying my day-pack when I set the record."

"I know," I said. "But we pay him well." I extended another doughnut hole to my hiking partner as he laughed and accepted the offering. Then we headed back into the woods together.

A few hours later, Dutch and I came out at a road crossing and met Brew. He had picked up blackberry milkshakes for the two of us, and also stopped at the drugstore to buy some antinausea medicine.

I sat down in my camp chair and started working on my milkshake.

"Brew, do you think Horton is acting weird?"

"What do you mean?" Brew replied. "Horton always acts weird."

"Well, in 2008, he kept saying things to me like, 'You're doing it, girl!' and 'This is really special!' And this summer he hasn't said anything like that."

"Well, in 2008 you weren't three days ahead of his old record."

"Yeah, but he always said before this summer that he thought I could set the overall record and that he wanted to help."

"He *does* want to help," Brew confirmed. "But he wants to be on the trail with you, and he can't keep up because he's tired and his knee hurts. He also wants you to run, and you're not running. The problem isn't that he doesn't want to help; the problem is he feels like he can't."

"Well, his doughnut holes are helpful."

Brew smiled. "Don't worry about Horton. His heart is in the right place. I know he would do anything in his power to help you."

The next day, our second in Shenandoah National Park, Horton proved his devotion.

I woke up feeling nauseous for the fifth straight morning, but this time it was even more overwhelming, and it was difficult to breathe. At five a.m., I took a few steps to the exact spot where I had stopped hiking the night before, then I turned around to look at Brew.

Instead of walking forward, I hiked backward toward him. For the first time since Vermont, I decided that I couldn't start hiking at five a.m. I felt absolutely horrible. All I wanted to do—all I was able to do—was sit down with my head between my legs. I tried to take deep breaths for several minutes, but they sounded labored, as if I had asthma. Brew stroked my back.

"Honey, do you want to lie down? Or what about putting your hands over your head? Or maybe you should drink something. Would that help?"

Brew was at a loss. And so was I. It felt like there was a cinder block on my chest. I knew that in that moment I couldn't hike. I laid down beside Brew and put both hands on my forehead. My breathing gradually became less labored, and as it did, my eyelids grew heavy. I dozed for the next hour or so, and then when I felt like I couldn't afford to rest any longer, I looked at Brew and said, "I need to get up."

He helped me to a sitting position and I felt okay. Then he took my hands and pulled me to my feet. At that point I felt really sick, but I knew that I couldn't afford to rest any longer.

Brew grabbed my gear, and together we went back to the same trailhead where I'd turned around an hour ago.

I looked back at my husband one more time.

"Do you need anything special?" he asked. "Can I get you some more medicine? What about doughnut holes?"

I hesitated. "I think what you should get me is a pregnancy test." And with that, I turned around and trudged off into the woods.

I didn't *really* think I was pregnant. I mean, I had taken the typical precautions to ensure that I wouldn't be. But I had never felt such severe nausea and exhaustion in my life. For the past three days, I had been contemplating whether or not birth control was still effective on a person who was hiking fifty miles and eating 6,000 calories per day. I highly doubted that the pharmaceutical company had run that research study.

I had always wanted to be a mom, but I was *not* ready to be pregnant!

I knew that if I took a pregnancy test and it came back positive, I would have to end my hike. Even though my ob-gyn was extremely progressive, I didn't think anyone would tell me that I could keep trudging so many miles per day if I was pregnant. Just like the non-existent birth control study, I was equally sure that there was not a test group for pregnant women hiking repeated fifty-mile days.

I had overcome so much, dealt was such adversity. It was strange and bittersweet to think that my hike could actually come to a halt because of something positive. I wanted to keep hiking, I wanted to do my best and finish the trail in less than forty-seven days. But in the grand scheme of things, if I had to pick between being a record holder and being a mother, then hands down, I wanted babies. I was convinced that being a mom was better and probably harder than any record, but I also hoped that starting a family could wait just a little bit longer.

I did the math. I had been on the trail for four weeks without having my monthly cycle, and I began to think of times that Brew and I had been intimate since leaving Katahdin. Thankfully, that wasn't too hard to keep track of.

In 2008, Brew and I began our hike twelve days after we were married. Thus, we "celebrated" our newlywed status nearly every night. When calculating all the ways I was going to add mileage this summer, I decided that foregoing sex would equal at least one extra mile per day. A half mile's worth of time plus a half mile's worth of energy equals one mile. It was all very scientific.

However, there were times on the trip where I needed the physical connection with Brew because it provided added emotional strength. For his part, Brew always claimed that it was probably one of the best ways I could stretch. "Think of it as multi-tasking," he would say. So yes, based on a few nights of stretching, it was not probable that I was knocked up, but it *was* possible.

The silver lining of needing to take a pregnancy test was that Brew was not the one who bought it. That honor had been bestowed upon Horton.

He and Dutch had stayed at a hotel in town, and Brew called and asked him to pick up the test on his way to the trail. I could just see our extremely conservative, self-aware, sixty-two-year-old friend walking into a drugstore to buy a pregnancy test. Man, what I wouldn't pay to get my hands on the surveillance video at *that* CVS! The mental image itself was priceless, and it helped take my mind off the potential life-altering implications. Brew was right; Horton would do just about anything to help us out.

The other piece of encouragement that kept my mind off the miles—and the possibility of having to quit—was that during my first two hours of hiking, I had seen seven bears. I often referred to the Shenandoah National Park as the Shenandoah Petting

Zoo. Deer graze inside the campgrounds, turkeys parade down the asphalt roads, and you have a better chance of spotting a bear in there than almost anywhere else on the trail. But seven bears before breakfast was unheard of!

Brew, Horton, and Dutch met me at Big Meadows Campground. They handed me a hot breakfast from the nearby lodge, and Horton handed me a brown bag.

I ate only a few bites of food, but this time it was due more to nerves than to nausea. Then I stood up and put the brown bag in my daypack.

"Do you want me to hike with you?" asked Dutch.

I smiled and replied, "I think I'd better do this section on my own." Then I leaned over and gave Brew a peck on the cheek.

"I'll see you in a few miles," I said.

For my husband, I am sure those were the longest miles of the entire trail. We hadn't had the opportunity to talk about it, and based on the look of uncertainty that crossed his face, I couldn't tell if he was excited, upset, or simply amused.

After leaving my crew, I hiked a little farther and then stepped into the woods to unwrap the pee stick. After doing my part to activate the test strip, I stood there hypnotized by the hourglass that kept flashing on the screen. My heart was racing. What was taking so long? Did Horton buy a faulty test? I could have been another quarter mile down the trail by now! But what would that even matter if I had to stop at the next road?

I decided to keep hiking with the test in my hand so I didn't waste any more time. Every day of this record attempt, I had wished for a valiant excuse to end the hike and stop the pain. Yet every day, I also prayed that nothing would force me to quit. Now my entire fate rested on a urine-saturated device that was clutched in the same hand as my hiking pole.

I waited for what seemed like an eternity. Finally, two words popped up: "Not Pregnant."

YES! Hallelujah. Thank you, Jesus. I had never felt so relieved.

I pumped my fist and my hiking stick in the air. But as my arm came down, I also began to feel a little bit—just ever so slightly, kind of, sort of—disappointed. I didn't want to be pregnant right then, but I decided that I would not be upset if that was the last negative pregnancy test I ever took.

At the next road crossing, I was surprised that Brew and Horton also seemed to respond to the test results with mixed emotions.

"Did you really think you were pregnant?" asked Horton.

"Well, I have never felt this nauseous, tired, and weak in my entire life. So yeah, I thought it was a possibility."

"Well, I'm glad that we don't have to quit the record attempt," said Brew, with a somewhat sullen look on his face. "You had better keep going. You have to make up for lost time this morning."

I looked straight at my husband. I heard what he was saying with his lips, but I also saw what he was communicating with his eyes. We both had a bad habit of planning our next adventure before we finished the one we were on. And after this morning, it was becoming very clear what that next adventure would be.

Dutch seemed to be the only person on our crew who was completely, one hundred percent happy that the test results were negative.

"Does this mean we can hike now?" he asked enthusiastically.

That afternoon, he and I waded through another thunderstorm, and that night I followed the back of his shoes with my headlamp until we arrived at our campsite. We had seen another seven bears since that morning. Fourteen bears in one day—now, that's a record!

When I made it to the first road south of Shenandoah National Park, Brew congratulated me with some more positive numbers.

"Guess how many miles you hiked last week?" he insisted.

"I don't know. A lot."

"Over three hundred fifty!" I liked positive numbers, but Brew loved them. "That's greater than the driving distance between Asheville and Nashville (a trip we made frequently to visit Brew's parents). And you did it on foot!"

"Well, I had a lot of help," I responded. I put my hand on Brew's knee as a sign of appreciation.

"Yeah, about that . . ." Brew's voice trailed off along with his excitement.

"*What* about that?" I demanded as my soft grip now started to squeeze his thigh.

"It's just that, you know Dutch is leaving in a day and a half, right?"

"Yeah, we've known that since Pennsylvania."

"Well, Horton is going to take him to the bus station and then he's going home, too."

"*What?*" I shrieked. "Horton's supposed to be here until the end of the trail! Why is he leaving?"

"You know why he's leaving," countered Brew. "He's not helping us on *his* terms, and we are going after this record on *our* terms. He's tired and hurt, and he needs to go home to be with his family."

"But *we're* supposed to be his family right now."

"It'll be okay. I'll find other people to come help us."

I felt a lump in my throat, and I swallowed hard to keep it down. "Well, I don't want to talk to him about it," I said.

"What do you mean?" asked Brew.

I wanted Horton to be where he wanted to be, and in my core I knew that he needed to be at home with his family. But it was still a broken promise, and it still hurt. I let go of Brew's leg and wiped a tear from my eye.

"It is really helping me to have him here. If he tells me he's leaving, I am going to cry, and I don't have the strength right now to deal with that."

"Okay," agreed Brew. "I'll let him know." Then he gently ran his fingers through my hair. I reached for his other hand and placed it against my cheek. "It'll be okay," he said. "*I'll* be here until the end. I promise."

The disappointment I felt when I found out Horton was leaving did not negate the fact that he had been a helpful part of our team for five full days. I was thankful for every moment that he'd spent with us. And then there was Dutch. He had helped for ten days now, and he had hiked roughly two-hundred-fifty miles with me. He'd become a fantastic hiking partner and friend.

Dutch was planning a visit to Washington, DC, before he had to return home. For a full forty-eight hours, Brew and I both tried to convince him that the nation's capital was overrated and that the free museums on the National Mall were not *that* special. We were only joking, of course, but we wouldn't have argued with Dutch if he'd decided to stay.

On his final night, he and I hiked over Three Ridges together. He laughed as I choked down a berry and Nutella burrito and then wiped the remaining chocolate spread all over my white-and-yellow shirt. On the backside of the mountain, we watched the sky light up in orange, then pink, and finally purple. Then we put our headlamps on, switched positions, and I followed the back of his dirt-covered shoes downhill to the Tye River.

At one point, we heard a small animal move right beside the trail. The unexpected sound made me instinctively leap ahead. I landed a few inches behind Dutch and grabbed his arm to regain my balance.

"What was that? A rabbit?" he asked.

"Nuh-uh, that wasn't a rabbit sound," I said.

I turned my head and looked back until my headlight located the brown-and-beige coil and flickering tongue just inches from the trail.

"What kind of snake is that?" asked Dutch.

"A copperhead," I replied. (Just the day before, I had introduced Dutch to his first rattlesnake.)

"You know," said Dutch, "I have seen more snakes, bears, sunrises, and sunsets with you in the past week and a half than on my entire thru-hike."

I smiled. "That's one of the best parts of trying to set a record," I said. "When the animals start to come out and the other hikers go to bed, we are still out here taking it all in."

Together, Dutch and I came to the banks of the Tye River just before ten p.m. Brew already had our tent set up, and after submerging myself in the nearby water, I climbed inside and ate dinner. Dutch came over to our tent and left something outside. Then without saying a word, I heard his nimble footsteps fade away.

I unzipped my flap and saw his elastic ankle braces resting near my shoes. My feet had been twisting and turning a lot recently and my ankles felt weak. Dutch knew I was uncomfortable, and he left me the same ankle braces he'd worn for his entire hike.

I pulled the worn, dirt-smeared sleeves into the tent. I examined them and then pulled the left one over my foot to see if it fit. *Perfect.* I started to slide it off my foot when a thought crossed my mind: If I could keep Dutch's ankle braces, then perhaps some of his superpowers would remain with me. Maybe now I would be able to night hike over three miles per hour on my own! I decided that I was going to wear those supports on every rocky stretch between the Tye River and Springer Mountain. Regardless of whether they were a source of superpower or superstition, they reminded me of good times and a good friend.

In return, I asked Brew to present Dutch with several bags of Combos, some Clif Bars, and any other items that now caused me to gag.

The next morning at 4:45 a.m., I woke up and crawled out of my tent to see Dutch's headlamp shining near the trail. Together, we hiked up the steep slope of the Priest. Just after summiting, we came to a road where Brew and Horton were waiting for us. I gave Dutch a long embrace, then reluctantly let go. I nodded my head at Horton and walked over to Brew. Dutch got into Horton's truck and soon all that was left of my two friends was a cloud of dust rising from a gravel road. I leaned on my husband as I watched them drive away.

· 12 ·

REINFORCEMENTS

JULY 14, 2011—JULY 21, 2011

As much as I wanted companionship on the trail, it was comforting and intimate to be only with my husband at the road crossings. There were certainly times when the two of us had been alone this summer, particularly if we had two support vehicles and different crew members meeting me at alternating trailheads. But the majority of our time had been spent with other people. Now, without additional helpers, the road crossings felt less frenetic and more honest. Brew and I both knew our roles and what needed to happen at the car; we didn't have to communicate that to each other or coordinate with the crew. And when we did talk, we said more with less.

"How do you feel?" he asked.

"Like shit," I said with a smile.

Brew laughed. "That makes sense." Then he paused thoughtfully, "I can't believe we're here."

I nodded my head in agreement. I knew exactly what he meant by "here." He meant home. We were finally in the Blue Ridge Mountains. We were an hour away from Charlottesville, Virginia, where we had gotten married, and we were crisscrossing paths where we had run ultra-races and gone on day hikes in the past. From this point forward, the mountains and terrain felt familiar. It was hard to believe that in a few more days we would enter Tennessee and North Carolina, and that after that we just had another seventy-five miles in Georgia until we reached the end. It was one of the first times that we had both allowed ourselves to think about it. But the thought didn't last long.

"Well, you'd better get going," said Brew.

I silently stood up and took my daypack out of his hand then gave him a kiss on the lips and walked toward the trail. Before I climbed the wooden stile over the barbed-wire fence that separated the road from the forest, I looked back at my husband.

"You know, Horton might not have said it this summer, but this *is* really special."

Brew smiled. "I know."

In a way, even though Horton wasn't with us, he still kept his promise to provide support until the end of the trail. He's one of the most connected ultra-runners in the world, and after he left, he arranged for several members of his tight-knit trail community to come out and help. The first person to join us after Horton's departure was Rebekah Trittipoe.

Rebekah is a tremendous athlete and ultra-running veteran. She was also the first female I'd hiked with since Melissa left in northern Pennsylvania. It was refreshing to share the trail with another woman. I needed some girl talk.

From the time I started backpacking years ago, most of my hiking partners have been men. I know far more than I care to recount concerning jock itch and male chafing (both below the belt and around the nipples). Men are not the only ones on the trail with issues, but conversation about female medical concerns still feels unacceptable in mixed company. In fact, if you ever want to lose a male hiking partner, I recommend broaching the subject of menstrual cramps or yeast infections.

Rebekah could not only relate to my issues, but she could also share war stories from hundred-mile races and multiday fast-packing trips. She told me tales of her seven-day race through the Amazon rain forest, of surviving the stinging nettles and rocks on the Allegheny Trail, and of running dozens of Horton's trail races.

Rebekah also shared stories from her path as a wife and mother. She was farther down that trail than I was, and I appreciated the advice she gave concerning the sharp turns and tough climbs that lay ahead. Above all, my favorite conversations with Rebekah centered around faith.

Rebekah was the first Christian I had been able to hike with all summer. One of the aspects I loved most about the Appalachian Trail community was its diversity of backgrounds and beliefs. But it was also nice to be honest and authentic with someone and not have them look at you like you're crazy.

I understand that a religion like Christianity that is based on a man who died (then came back to life) 2,000 years ago seems far-fetched and radical. I also understand that I am a member of a religion that has had a hand in numerous wars and unspeakable tragedies. For a rational person, faith in a belief system like this can seem completely illogical. Which is why it's really nice to just share it sometimes and not always have to explain it.

"So do you pray while you hike?" asked Rebekah.

"Yeah, all the time. But I spend so much time in my head that sometimes it's nice to just listen."

"What do you think God is telling you?"

"That I am supposed to be here. Not necessarily that I'm going to set a record, but that somehow, in some way, this is part of his plan for my life."

"Don't you wish that sometimes God picked easier plans?"

I laughed. "Yeah, that would be nice."

"Well, what do you think God is teaching you through all this?" she asked.

"Trust. He's definitely teaching me about trust," I said. "And dependence. I need him more than ever out here." I paused for a few seconds. "And also, I think I am learning to live in the present instead of worrying about tomorrow. Oh, and he's teaching me about love. I am learning a heck of a lot about love."

"What do you mean?"

"Well, the other night Brew told me that the reason he's out here being so supportive and loving is because he feels like it's his responsibility as a Christian husband. He mentioned the Bible verse where God calls men to love their wives like Christ loved the church. Out here, Brew is willing to sacrifice himself to love me well, and it's making me fall more in love with him and more in love with Christ."

Rebekah nodded her head. "You're *really* lucky. Most men don't understand just how manly unselfishness really is."

All of the crew members had helped me physically and emotionally, but it was really nice to have someone like Rebekah to encourage me spiritually. Being with her reminded me of why Brew and I had set out on this journey. The purpose wasn't to impress anyone, but simply to praise and delight an audience of One.

Despite being a runner, Rebekah spent three of her four nights with us carrying a full backpack for me. And watching a runner carry a backpack is almost as painful as watching a fish flop around on dry ground. It's just awkward and out of place. I will admit, though, that after carrying a light daypack and having people "mule" me for several weeks, I didn't fare much better.

The first night wasn't so bad. We decided that we would camp near the James River, but we crossed it after dark and couldn't find where Brew had set up camp. With his ACL tear, he was limited to hiking no more than a quarter mile, and after we traveled twice that distance, we still hadn't seen him.

Rebekah handed her pack to me. She had picked up her overnight gear and some extra food at our car, which was parked near the James River footbridge. In my exhaustion, the pack felt as if it were filled with bricks. I sat on the trail and started rummaging through her bag, looking for snacks while she backtracked to see if we had passed Brew unknowingly in the darkness.

Finally, after about fifteen minutes and a few dozen vanilla wafers, I heard someone hiking toward me, and I called out, "Hello?! Brew? Rebekah?"

"It's me," my husband responded as his headlamp appeared through the trees.

"What happened? Where have you been? Where's the tent?"

"It's just a little farther," he said. "I was making such good time that I accidentally hiked more than I was supposed to."

I couldn't decide whether to be happy that his knee was feeling good or suspicious that he was trying to increase my mileage for the day.

The next evening, after a long, hot day that started just south of the James River, I found myself crisscrossing the Blue Ridge Parkway near Roanoke. I'd hiked up and down steep mountains all morning and afternoon, and now my legs and chest felt weak. I knew that I had another twelve miles, almost entirely downhill, until I would reach the outskirts of Troutville.

I'd already put in forty miles, and I didn't know if I had another twelve in me. Brew suggested that he could meet me at a forest service road after another six miles. There, if I wanted to, I could collect my backpacking gear and hike a few more miles before camping out in the forest.

I enjoyed the gentle descent off the parkway, but after a few miles, the trail started undulating up and down steep inclines. Where did these hills come from? And why were they so hard?!

The only two things I remembered about this section from previous journeys was that once I had seen a bear here, and the other time, I had hiked while watching the sunset. Why didn't I remember all this climbing? It was as if someone had just put these hills on the trail within the past two years. Up down, up down, up down. My calves burned and my thighs quivered. When I reached the overgrown forest-service road where Brew was waiting for me, I was completely spent.

I sat down and he handed me my dinner—spaghetti stuffed inside a tortilla wrap. A look of disgust came over my face, though I knew full well I'd brought this upon myself.

Since leaving Maine, I'd asked my husband for foods that I could hold. Small finger foods or anything requiring a utensil took too much time and attention. But at this moment, my need to feel civilized outweighed my desire to be efficient. I refused to eat spaghetti inside of a burrito. Even a hiker had to draw the line somewhere. So I unwrapped the tortilla and buried my face in the noodles like a pig at a trough. That's dignity for you.

While I worked on slurping up my dinner, Brew filled my large overnight pack with a tent, sleeping bag, nightclothes, more food, and more water. He also included a large foot-care kit with disinfectant, Vaseline, powder, corn cushions, athletic tape, and clean socks. After wiping the marinara sauce off my face with a Wet One, I stood up and put on my pack.

In reality, it weighed no more than twenty pounds, but it felt like a hundred. I adjusted the straps, but it still felt like a wooden yoke resting on my shoulders. Once I'd walked forty or fifty yards, Brew called.

"There isn't any camping out near Troutville, so I'll probably get a hotel room tonight in Roanoke. If you make good time, maybe I can take you back there in the morning for a quick shower."

"Okay. Love you," I yelled back. Then I kept walking.

My pace decreased significantly due to the pack weight. I thought about Brew. Then I thought about the hotel room.

After hiking just over a mile, I started to whimper and my eyes felt damp. I had been so tough for most of this trip. But in this moment I felt like a wimp, a wimp who wanted sympathy. I took out my cell phone and called Brew.

As soon as he picked up, I wailed, "I wanna stay in the hotel, *too*!"

"What did you say?" asked Brew. "What's wrong? Are you okay?" The reception was bad, so he was yelling.

I wiped my snotty nose with my forearm, leaving dirt streaks from my elbow to my wrist, then I tried again.

"I want to stay in the hotel, *too*. I want to take a shower tonight and sleep in a clean bed with *you*. Carrying a pack was a BAD idea! I should have just hiked to the next road." I took a deep breath, then finished on a shrill note, emphasizing the last few words as each came out: "This is an *inefficient—use—of—my—energy!*"

Then I started whimpering again.

"Look up," said Brew.

I lifted my head and rubbed my eyes. He was standing about fifty yards ahead.

Suddenly, I no longer felt the pack pressing into my shoulders or weighing down my legs. I started jogging.

"Slow down. Don't fall!" he said.

But I was afraid if I didn't get to him fast enough, he might disappear.

I threw my arms around his neck.

"What are you doing here?" I asked.

"Well, I saw a short side trail by the road when I was driving up here earlier. I thought it probably led to the trail, but I didn't want to tell you about it in case I was wrong and I didn't get to see you again."

"I don't want to camp out anymore," I sobbed.

Brew smiled. "Yeah, I gathered."

Then he offered a solution.

"I can take your pack, but that means you won't get down to the road until close to eleven p.m. If you get in that late and stay at the hotel with me, I still want you to get six hours of sleep. So you can't start until five thirty or six in the morning. Is that a deal?"

I slung the pack off my shoulders and laid it at Brew's feet. Just then, we saw Rebekah hiking toward us. She had started at the road near Troutville and hiked in to camp with me. We told her about the change of plans, and she happily unloaded her overnight gear on Brew, as well. Then Brew left us, and together we continued downhill. The only upside of temporarily carrying a pack was that once it was off, I felt like I was drifting effortlessly down the trail.

The hotel and shower were worth the late night and the extra miles, but the next evening I found myself in a similar predicament. It became clear that Rebekah and I would have to pack in together and camp out on the trail if I wanted to achieve my target mileage. After my whinefest the night before, we decided that Rebekah would hike in ahead of me, carrying a pack with all our gear. All I would have to do is wear my daypack and catch up with her.

I said good-bye to Brew at dusk and hiked into the forest to find Rebekah. Within a few minutes, I had to turn on my headlamp. After spending so many dark hours walking with Dutch and after receiving his ankle braces, I was now a more confident night hiker. But beyond Craig Creek Valley, the A.T. proved hard to follow. There were multiple times when I thought I was on the right path and then discovered that I was lost in a maze of rhododendron trees.

It took me longer than I'd expected to find Rebekah, which made me worry that she or I—or both of us—was lost. When I finally did see her, it was clear she was struggling under the weight of the pack. She looked like a spinning top wobbling out of control. We'd planned on camping at a spring near the ridge, but at the rate Rebekah was traveling, it would have taken us a long time to get there.

"Rebekah, let me carry the pack," I said.

"No, you're not carrying the pack. That's my job."

"You've already carried it most of the way. It's my pack and it doesn't fit you well. Trust me, we can go faster if I carry it."

She still refused, and we continued slowly in the dark. After a long while, we realized that even though our pace was sluggish, we still should have arrived at the water source. The darkness and decreased pace had me feeling disoriented. I could no longer sense how far we had come or how far we had to go to reach the spring. Then a light rain began to fall.

By this point, we were on a rocky ridge where the path was becoming slick and dangerous. Between the two of us, we had only a few sips of water left. Still, we decided that as soon as we found a flat spot, we would stop and set up the tent. It was too risky to keep going or look for a water source.

Five minutes later, the trail offered a small level shoulder, and we stopped to set up camp. I was so thirsty that I honestly thought about licking the outside of the tent to lap up some of the moisture that had collected on the thin fabric. Instead, I drank a protein shake that Brew had packed with my dinner, and I went to bed feeling parched. Rebekah, on the other hand, went to bed without drinking anything and saved our few remaining sips of water so I could wet my mouth in the morning.

"Rebekah," I protested, "you need to drink something. Just finish it. I'll be fine. I promise."

"There is no way I am drinking that water," she said. "You have to hike fifty miles tomorrow. I have to hike five miles, downhill, to my car, and then I am going home. You need it more than I do."

I was going to miss Rebekah. She was refreshing in so many ways.

The next morning, I drank a swig of water, said good-bye to Rebekah, and left the tent at five a.m. It was six miles to the next road crossing. As soon as I arrived, I walked over to our filthy car, opened our trunk, and was immediately struck by the smell of dirty, wet socks. I grabbed some water and juice and started to chug. Brew was still in the tent a few yards away, and it looked like he was cleaning the ground cloth with soap and water. As was evidenced by the inside and outside of our car, it's not in my husband's nature to clean, and it certainly isn't in his nature to scrub.

So I asked, "What are you doing?"

"Well . . . something funny happened last night," he said coyly.

"What was that?" I asked between gulps of fruit juice and water.

"Um, I think a groundhog peed on our tent," he said.

"What?" I exclaimed.

Then he looked at me with a sheepish smile, and I started laughing. I quickly figured out what had happened. I could see that Brew had camped on a slope. He always took a bathroom

break at night, and last night he must have peed uphill. Our poor
tent! Everything we had—our car, our gear, our bodies—it all told
the story of the past 1,500 miles.

"Where are we now? How many miles do we have left?" I asked.
It was meant as a rhetorical joke. But when I thought about it, I
wasn't sure I wanted to know the answer.

After Rebekah left, Brew and I enjoyed another stretch of private
meetings on forest service roads and asphalt. Usually when we
thru-hiked together, we would experience our worst arguments
during the first week of the trip. After that, things would usually
be very harmonious and agreeable, until the "almost-end." The
almost-end is one of the hardest parts of any journey. It comes
at the point when you are more uncomfortable, tired, and weak
than you have been since you began, but you are too far from the
finish to feel hopeful.

You are waiting for your second wind, for the motivation you
need to bypass fatigue and accomplish your goal. Brew and I had
avoided our usual fallout in the first week, and now I was hoping
to prevent the almost-end argument as well. So I decided to do a
little preventative maintenance.

"Do you know where we are?" I asked Brew.

"On a dirt road in southwest Virginia," he answered.

"Yes, and do you know approximately how many more days we
have to reach Springer?" I had done the math, and I was confident
that Brew had too. In fact, he even had his "positive numbers pen"
in hand. Most of the time he used it to calculate my mileages on
a clipboard, but currently he was doodling a smiley face on my
thigh.

"If you stay on schedule, then we have less than two weeks to
go," he said.

"That's right. You have done such an *amazing* job this summer, and I want to make sure that I am extra kind and appreciative toward you this week." I said all of this in my most syrupy-sweet voice. "And it would really help me if for the next few days you could be even *more* encouraging and supportive than you usually are."

"Ahhh . . ." Brew knew where I was headed. "We are at the almost-end, aren't we?"

I nodded.

"Yeah." He hesitated, then went on, "I don't know what else I have to give, and I don't know how you can keep doing what you are doing, but we both need to find more. So let's try to find it together." Then he took his pen and began a new sketch near my knee.

"When do you think it's going to feel like the *real* end?" he asked.

"Erwin, Tennessee," I said. "I think when we get there and we only have a week left, it'll start to feel like—OWWW!" I wailed as Brew nearly punctured me in the quad with an exclamation mark.

I looked down at my leg. It now read "L-O-V-E-!"

"That hurt!" I cried.

"Love hurts," Brew said with a smirk.

My next trail companion was a legend among hikers and ultra-runners in the Southeast. Matt Kirk had hiked the Appalachian Trail twice and was the first person to run the hundred-mile stretch of the A.T. in Shenandoah National Park in less than twenty-four hours. He had set endurance records on the 1,000-mile Mountains-to-Sea Trail, the three-hundred-fifty mile Benton McKaye Trail, and the hundred-mile Bartram Trail, and he was also the fastest to string together all of the Southeastern peaks above 6,000 feet. We had never hiked together, and to put it lightly, I was a little intimidated.

Matt brought his wife Lily to join us. Lily was beautiful and kind, *and* an A.T. thru-hiker. Their relationship had been cemented on the trail's northernmost five hundred miles.

At this point, the efforts of my support crew had yielded thirty completions of the Appalachian Trail and over 65,000 miles of collective wisdom and experience. More than ever, I was convinced that this journey was anything but a solo effort.

Matt and I set out together from Wind Rock. Our plan was to meet Brew and Lily twenty-six miles later at the Senator Shumate Bridge in Pearisburg, Virginia. We were accompanied on the trail by his mutt Uwharrie. Uwharrie was also a thru-hiker. (Correction: the collective wisdom and experience of *thirty-one* A.T. completions now carried me down the trail.)

If I had to guess, I would say most dogs I know would prefer the couch and an unending bowl of dog food to the rough footing and relentless miles of the A.T. I had come across one too many dogs with shredded footpads and clearly defined rib cages to ever consider having a pet join me. However, Uwharrie and Matt were simpatico. You could tell that nothing made either of them happier than hiking down the trail.

Because Matt had set several trail records himself, I didn't have to begin our discourse by explaining why I wanted to hike the A.T. this way. And he didn't ask me if it was fun, because he already knew that it wasn't. Just as Rebekah and I understood each other's faith, Matt and I both understood trail records. And instead of explaining our choices, we spent time defending them.

"I think one of the main problems is not that people misunderstand trail records," I said. "It's that they misunderstand traditional backpacking. I took nearly five months on my first A.T.

thru-hike, and until now, it has been the most difficult of all my hikes. I don't care if you are hiking ten miles a day or fifty, the trail is still hard, you're still going to get eaten by bugs, and you're still going to feel dirty and tired. Anyone who expects hiking to be perpetually comfortable and fun is probably a day hiker who travels non-technical trails in good weather."

"Yeah, I feel you," said Matt. "I usually think that the harder a hike is, the greater the reward. Between my relationship and my job, I can't backpack as much as I used to. Putting in big miles lets me get my fill—and stay married and employed. It also allows me to draw more strength from nature. I remember one time on the Long Trail, I had just given my last piece of food to Uwharrie going up Camel's Hump, and I was starving and frustrated with myself for not carrying enough supplies. But then I arrived at the summit and the view was so awesome that I drew energy from it. I just drank it in, and, man, I just started cruising down the trail. It was almost like I was floating."

I felt like Matt was floating down the trail right now, gliding in front of me with his long, steady strides. Like Dutch, Matt was one of the few people I hiked with who had longer legs than I did. I was working hard to keep up, and Uwharrie made it worse by constantly running between us, reminding me that he was actually hiking twice as far as his two-legged companions.

"Matt, do you mind if I hike in front for a while?"

"Of course not. Do whatever you need to do. The entire reason I am out here is to help you."

I was still a little overwhelmed by Matt's trail resume and his hiking skills, but it helped that he was as mellow and supportive as he was accomplished.

When Matt and I reached the bridge, Brew's jaw dropped.

"I didn't think you guys would be here for at least another hour!" he exclaimed. "You were hiking almost four miles per hour."

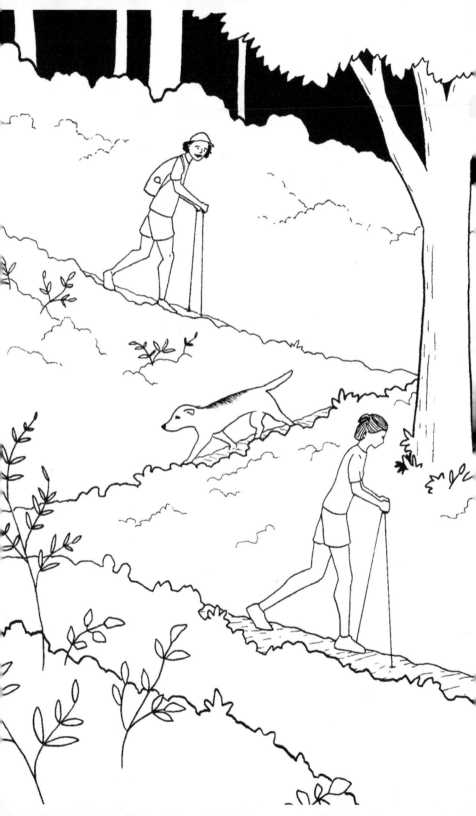

I smiled. I knew that I could not have hiked as quickly or en-joyed that section as much without Matt. Unfortunately, he was not willing to take the 4:45 a.m. shift the following morning. He was, after all, a teacher on summer vacation. But then again, so was my husband.

The next morning, Brew and I walked through Pearisburg in the dark, then I started hiking alone toward Angel's Rest. The sun had not come up yet and it was already sweltering. I was pouring sweat, my clothes were clinging to my skin, and the air was so thick that it was hard to swallow. At least, having grown up in the South, I was somewhat accustomed to these conditions. I considered my roots a real advantage on the record. It would have been difficult, if not impossible, to tolerate the heat and humidity otherwise.

Matt rejoined me on the next section, and that helped take my mind off of the high temperatures for a while. However, that afternoon, we were reminded of the summer swelter in a most unpleasant way when we came across deer carcasses lying near two separate road crossings.

Throughout the entire trip, I had refused to take extra steps.

I always wanted Brew to park exactly at the road crossing, and if there wasn't room on the shoulder of the road, then I expected him to park nearby and carry all the supplies to the trail. (I know, it sounds ridiculous. But my husband had told me it was okay to be a diva, so I was.) Sometimes the distance between the car and the trail was only twenty yards, but that was still twenty yards too far. I'd decided that if I had to hike over forty-six miles per day, then I wasn't going to waste any of my energy by walking off-trail.

However, in this scenario, the stench at the road crossing was so unbearable that I had no choice but to walk up the road and upwind. Matt had to go even farther, as Lily had refused to park within two hundred yards of the rotting flesh. Ever since hitting Maryland, the thought of a Clif Bar had made me gag, so you can imagine what the smell of a decaying animal did to me. I had only thrown up once on this trip, and I didn't want to repeat the experience. As soon as I started dry heaving, I just grabbed the snacks out of Brew's hands and raced down the trail.

I wasn't grossed out by the dead animal—the smell, yes, but not the animal. I was really frustrated and angry at the person who dumped it there. What a waste! There wasn't a single part of the body that had been used. It wasn't hunting season, and I assumed that a poacher had killed simply for sport. Three hundred years ago, Native Americans and settlers would have used the meat for food, the skin for clothing, the sinew for string, and the bones for tools. Now we have a tendency to treat our natural resources like garbage.

The next road crossing was similarly unpleasant. As the smell grew stronger, so did my nausea and my frustration. The only one who didn't seem to mind the putrid scent was Uwharrie. I was utterly impressed with that dog's olfactory senses. Not only had he detected the carcasses well before Matt or I had, but when we came to a junction with an intersecting path, Uwharrie always headed down the right trail without missing a step. He must have been following the scent of previous thru-hikers—which is almost as bad as that of a dead deer.

As the sun started to go down, I relied more on Uwharrie than on my headlamp. And as Matt and I headed down to our final road crossing, we resumed our conversation about trail records.

"Matt, do you ever think you would want to try for an A.T. record?"

"I don't know," he said. "I think if I tried for a record on the A.T., I would probably go after Ward Leonard's sixty-day unsupported record. I love the idea of being self-sufficient. But the most time I have ever spent going after a record was twenty-four days on the Mountains-to-Sea Trail, and I don't know if my body could handle that type of effort for two months."

Matt paused for a moment, then asked, "What does it feel like trying to set a 2,181-mile record?"

I thought about his question for a minute, then answered, "Well, it feels like I'm breaking down."

I continued, "Initially I thought there might be a turning point where my body would adjust or adapt to the challenge, but that never happened. Not on this challenge, anyway. There's been no time to rest or recover. So from the second I started, I've been experiencing a physical and emotional decline. I think the key to setting a record out here is just to try and break down as slowly and intelligently as possible, without completely shattering."

When we arrived at the road, I was relieved to find we weren't camping next to another dumpsite for poachers. Instead, we were treated to one of our best nights of the entire summer. Our tent was buried beneath a thicket of rhododendron beside Laurel Creek. I washed off in the clear, cool water underneath a dark sky full of twinkling white stars. Then I crawled into my tent to eat rehydrated sweet-and-sour chicken. And while I ate, I was serenaded by the sound of crickets, southern katydids, and the swirling currents of the nearby stream.

The campsite was perfect. There was a cool breeze, running water, humming insects, and soft black dirt to sleep on. The man I loved was nearby, and two friends were camped on the opposite riverbank. I was surrounded by life and beauty. My soul was content, and my life felt full. I thought about all the time Matt and I had spent discussing trail records over the past two days. In so many ways it did seem like trail records were similar to faith. You couldn't really explain it or make it make sense; you just had to experience it to appreciate its value.

The next morning, Matt and Lily left, and despite their tremendous contribution, I didn't bat an eyelash at their departure. I had one thing—or rather one person—on my mind. Hazel.

I love my husband, and I love my friends and family, but all those relationships require work. There was something about loving our nine-month-old niece that seemed effortless. As soon as she was born, she instantly captured my love and devotion. I'm guessing the feeling of being an aunt is only a shadow of what it's like to be a mother, and if that's the case I am in trouble, because I would do anything for my brother's little girl.

Amid the shin splints, diarrhea, nausea, and exhaustion, one of the toughest parts of trying to set a trail record was being away from Hazel. At home in Asheville, we only lived six miles apart, and I spent many training runs going back and forth to see her. Knowing that my brother James and sister-in-law Lindsay were coming to the trail with Hazel meant that I was light-footed and light-hearted all morning.

But within a mile of the road where I was planning to meet my family, my furious pace came to an abrupt stop. That was because ten feet away in the middle of the trail was a large timber rattlesnake. This was not my first rattlesnake of the summer, nor would it be my last, but it *was* the only one that refused to move. As soon as it saw me, it coiled into a tight circle and started shaking its tail so fast that it blurred.

I stood there and tapped my hiking poles against the earth because usually the vibrations cause snakes to slither away—but not this one. Then I picked up a few sticks and threw them near the snake. Still, it refused to relinquish its position. I looked to my right and left, but I was surrounded by a mountain laurel thicket, and getting off the path would mean crawling through a jungle gym of branches.

I tried to be polite and talk to him in a very soothing tone so that he would know I was not a threat.

"Hi, Mr. Snake," I said. "I would really appreciate it if you could slide off the trail now so I can keep going."

If anything, the rattler's tail seemed to speed up after my comment. Then my tone became less soothing.

"Listen here, you camouflaged belly-crawler, this trail is for foot traffic only! I've come over 1,500 miles to see my niece, and I'm not going to let you get between us now!"

With that I launched another stick, which landed a few inches away from the serpent. The poisonous blockade now reared its head and lifted its flickering tongue higher into the air. After several minutes, I realized it was not going to back down, so I stepped off-trail and began to weave and crawl through the maze of branches. The snake simply turned its head and kept shaking as I gave it a wide berth. The snake had won, and that didn't surprise me. Whenever I tried to enforce my will upon Mother Nature, she always won.

My attention soon shifted. When I heard the distant sound of a car, I quickened my pace and began yelling at the top of my lungs, "Hazel, Ha-zel!" Within minutes I came out to a clearing where Brew, James, and Lindsay sat with Hazel, who was crawling on a blanket. I immediately scooped up my niece. She did not seem to mind that I was damp to the touch and smelled horrible. She simply smiled, then showed off her newest developmental skill by clapping her hands. Perfect timing.

I sat down in my camp chair and put Hazel on her blanket. Brew put food in front of me. I knew I needed to eat, but all I wanted to do was play with my little niece. It seemed that she was hungry, too, because she kept trying to crawl off her blanket to grab handfuls of dirt and shove them in her mouth. I could already tell she was going to be a hiker.

As much as I wanted to play with Hazel on the blanket all day, Lindsay picked her up after fifteen minutes and took her to the car, but not before promising they would both be at the next road crossing. Getting to see Hazel again was the only motivation I needed to grab a pack and start striding down the trail, this time with my brother close behind me.

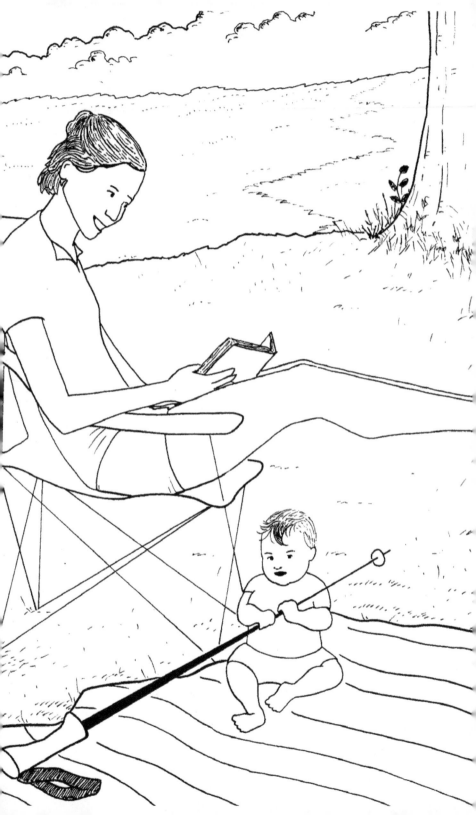

It was really nice to have James on the trail with me; not just because he could fill me in on all the cute things that Hazel had done over the past five weeks, but also because he was my brother. Getting my family to support my love of long-distance hiking had been a gradual and arduous process.

Eight years ago, James was not thrilled when I first set out alone at age twenty-one to hike the entire Appalachian Trail. But he was there at the end to climb Katahdin with me and help me drive home. Now he was back on the trail, trekking with me through the open fields and pastures of Southwest Virginia.

I appreciated his help, but in a way he owed me because I had spent my entire childhood going to every football, basketball, and baseball game that my brothers ever played—and their teams were never even that good. By the time I had my own tournaments and matches, both of my brothers were away at college, so they attended very few of my athletic events.

That afternoon, I asked James to fill me in on all the pro sports results I had missed over the summer. He told me about the NBA finals and gave me a brief recap of Wimbledon, then he asked me if I had heard about the U.S. Women's Soccer Team, which I, of course, had not.

"It was awesome!" he proclaimed. "They had an amazing run in the World Cup this summer. It felt like the entire country was rooting for them."

I had never heard my brother talk about women's soccer before.

So I asked, "Do you think you appreciate women's athletics more now that you have a daughter?"

"Yeah, I guess I do," he said reflectively. "I want Hazel to play any sport that she wants, and I hope she'll have other women to look up to."

"Yeah, I wish the media did a better job of portraying women as legitimate athletes," I added. "It makes me really mad how *Sports Illustrated* features men on the front cover all year until it is time for the swimsuit edition. What does that say to young girls? You have a better chance of landing a cover on *SI* by taking your top off than by excelling in an actual sport?"

I stopped talking, and James didn't respond. My brother has a quiet, pensive nature, which tends to make me more loquacious.

"It's not that I am against women being sex symbols," I continued—this conversation had started to get a little awkward, considering I was talking with my brother. "I am fine with men and women being sex symbols; we are all sexual creatures. I just want women to have the chance to be taken seriously as athletes, as well."

"Do you really feel like people give you less chance of setting the record because you're a woman?" asked James.

"*Of course* they do!" I responded. "In ultra-running, when a guy gets beaten by a women, he usually says that he got 'chicked.' It's common lingo at the finish line, and it implies that there is something inherently embarrassing about it. And I'm not arguing that most men aren't genetically stronger and faster than women, because that's a proven fact. But when it comes to endurance sports, the stronger, faster person doesn't always win."

"Well, I'm glad Hazel's going to have an aunt who's a terrific female athlete—no, wait. Strike that," James said. "I'm glad Hazel is going to have an aunt who is a terrific *athlete* to look up to."

Having Hazel join us on the trail for a day and a half boosted my mileage and my spirit. At the road crossings, Brew would keep an eye on his watch, and after ten minutes, he would lift our niece from my arms and tell me that I couldn't hold her again until the next road crossing.

At some point along the journey, another hiker had asked in a skeptical tone how I could prevent a passion from turning into an obsession. And I had answered that as long as I surrounded myself with people who loved me and held me accountable, I could give my all to this hike without worrying about compromising who I was. Brew and I both wanted to be good spouses, family members, and friends more than we wanted to set a trail record. I think the people who were closest to us knew that this hike only represented a season of our lives and did not ultimately define who we were. Knowing that probably made it easier for them to support our insane endeavor in the short term.

Hazel was a good reminder of where our priorities stood. But at the same time, her visit made me want to hike stronger and faster so that I could go home and be the best friend, sister, daughter, and aunt that I could be. Hazel *also* reinforced the growing notion that I wanted to finish so I could be a mom.

· 13 ·

LEANING HARD

JULY 21, 2011—JULY 26, 2011

When James, Lindsay, and Hazel left us, I was downtrodden, to say the least. As they departed, we were closing in on Damascus and the Virginia-Tennessee border. I should have been elated to leave behind the five-hundred twenty-five mile stretch of Virginia and to enter one of the last three states. But instead, I felt stuck.

When I met Brew at the next road crossing, he knew by my sullen look that something was wrong.

"You miss Hazel, don't you?"

"Yes," I said. "But I also hate where we are right now."

"You mean because it is still the almost-end?"

"Yeah. It's as if we are in trail purgatory," I replied. "I feel like I have given this trail everything, and I have made it a really long way, but I can sense that I am almost on empty and we are not anywhere close to the finish. I am hurting, and I am tired, and there is no end in sight."

"At least you know that," said Brew.

"What do you mean?"

"Well," Brew said, "you know this trail inside and out. And so far you have paced yourself perfectly. Someone else might try to give too much at this point because they think they're closer to the end than they really are. But you know every mountain, valley, and river between here and Springer, and I know that somewhere in your subconscious, you've kept enough strength in reserve to make it through the last five hundred miles."

I heard what Brew was saying, but it didn't help much. I was at a point on the trail where I really needed inspiration. Fortunately, I got what I needed when Maureen arrived.

Maureen was a life-long family friend, and she had been a small part of my first thru-hike in 2005 when I got off the trail in Hot Springs, North Carolina, to watch the NCAA men's basketball tournament at her house. During that visit, she prepared a huge dinner for me and a warm bucket of water with Epsom salts so I could eat, watch the game, and soak my sore feet all at the same time.

Maureen knew about endurance and efficiency. She was one of the toughest women I knew. When she was my age, she participated in a number of endurance riding events on horseback, including multiple hundred-mile rides in the back-country. Now in her sixties, she lived on a farm and trained her four border collies to participate in sheepdog trials—another sport where precision is key and the slightest mistake has huge consequences.

Whether at a national trial or at home, Maureen usually had two or three dogs trailing at her feet and an SLR camera hanging from her neck. She is the most gifted photographer I know. The only problem is that she refuses to shoot humans.

Maureen would capture images of sheep, dogs, and horses all day long, but she typically insisted that we two-legged creatures were not worth the trouble. It had been a three-month struggle to convince her to be our wedding photographer. For me, it wasn't just about having great photographs; it was about sharing such an intimate occasion with someone I knew and loved. Maureen finally agreed.

Not only did she take pictures at our outdoor wedding, but when a five-foot black snake crawled across the aisle just before the guests arrived, Maureen snatched it up by the head and slung it into the distant hedges.

Taking photos at our ceremony must not have been too unbearable, because two months after our nuptials, Maureen was also at Springer Mountain with her camera in hand as we set the women's supported record.

Usually she would have hiked a mile or more to get on-trail shots, but this summer she was limited to the road crossings. With her hair growing slower than Brew's beard, and a chest as flat as mine, we couldn't help but be reminded that Maureen had faced a journey much longer and more difficult than our own.

When we found out late last summer that Maureen had a progressive form of breast cancer, it surprised everyone. She was one of the strongest, fiercest women I knew. In a sense, we all felt that she was invincible. But last autumn, for the first time ever, I saw her cry. I wanted to give her something to look forward to, so I told her, even before telling my own parents, that I wanted to set the overall record on the trail and I wanted her to be there at the end to take photos. She looked at me and scoffed. And in her shrill Southern accent, she said, "I don't even know if I'll be *alive* next summer."

A few weeks into her treatment, Maureen and I went shopping together for only the second time. The first time had been when we were searching for my wedding dress; now we were looking for a wig. I watched as the thinning hair on her head was completely shaved off, and then helped her try on hairpieces of different lengths and colors. She ultimately decided she'd always wanted to be a redhead, so she chose a beautiful shoulder-length auburn coiffure. But that was the only day I ever saw her wear it. In the end, it didn't really suit her to wear a wig—or to have reconstructive breast surgery. There had never been anything artificial about Maureen.

In the past nine months, she had experienced a double mastectomy and multiple rounds of chemotherapy and radiation. Now, she was standing at the trailhead smiling, snapping pictures, and reminding me that when a task feels overwhelming, the only thing to do is take one step at a time. Maureen was an everyday hero. She was struggling and persevering because she had to, not because she wanted to. The grace and determination that she exhibited during her cancer treatment made me realize that I still had more to give, and it helped me to stop complaining. This endeavor was difficult, but I had *chosen* to be here and could stop at any time. Maureen's resolve was unwavering and her battle was ongoing. Her presence on the trail was humbling and inspiring, and her story and example helped me through the almost-end.

Often, when I arrived at a road crossing I would find Maureen and Brew bickering. Maureen gave both of us tough love, just like my mom would. It was great entertainment watching her chide my husband.

"You need to let me clean the inside of the car," she would nag. "It is an absolute mess! If you don't rinse out this cooler with soap and water, Jen is going to get a bacterial infection."

"Okay, okay, I'll do it," Brew would reply.

"No, you don't have time to do it. You need to let me help you."

"But you don't know where to look for things or what container to put them in."

"Oh, and you do? *Anything* would be better than the state this car is in right now."

Then Maureen looked over at me sitting in the camp chair.

"Oh my God, Momie! What is that you're putting in your mouth?"

Maureen has called me Momie since I was born. To this day, I don't know why, but just hearing the nickname makes me feel loved.

I'll admit, I had started to include French fries and a milkshake as one of my daily snacks. I also continued drinking fruit smoothies; squirting honey in my mouth; and eating healthy sandwiches, Greek yogurt, and guacamole as much as possible. But I was still extremely nauseous, and fries and a milkshake were still somewhat appetizing, and they went down easily.

"You can't set a record by eating French fries all the time! Here, I brought fruit and some hard-boiled eggs from my chickens."

Then she handed me several zipper-lock bags from the cooler in her truck bed. "You need to eat some of this, too," she said. I dug inside one of the bags and brought out a giant hunk of watermelon.

I filled my mouth with the sweet red flesh and let the juice run down my chin. It tasted delicious. I guess watermelon also worked pretty well as a trail snack. The only problem was I didn't have time to isolate the seeds in my mouth and spit them out so I just swallowed them. Watermelon may be healthier, but I never had to worry about seeds when I ate French fries.

"Keep that and eat it," said Maureen. "I'm going back to the farm tomorrow. I'll bring you some more fresh fruit toward the end of the trail."

When we reached the North Carolina border, things felt as if they had come full circle. I was in my home state, where I had grown up, and soon I reached the place where I'd first set foot on the Appalachian Trail.

Just north of Roan Mountain, I passed a rural county road near a cemetery and a church where on a day hike in 2004 I had seen my first white blaze. I passed by a familiar tree with a double blaze and laughed out loud. I remembered wondering eight years ago what on earth two off-set blazes could possibly mean. Now, I instinctively veered left, knowing the two white rectangles signified a sudden change of direction.

I loved walking over the top of Roan in the mid-morning mist and smelling the sweet scent of the Fraser fir and spruce trees that bordered the trail. This had been one of the portions of trail where I'd spent time training in the spring, and it was amazing how different it looked just two months later. The flame azalea and rhododendron no longer showcased their brilliant colors, but the green was deeper than I remembered and the scent of evergreen was stronger. I knew that I would smell this aroma again on Unaka Mountain and on the ridges of the Smokies—only two more high-elevation, Christmas-scented summits left.

When I reached the Nolichucky River, I was met by Brew and two of our best friends, Jeff and Heather. I could drive from our house to the Nolichucky River in less than an hour, so it was close enough for frequent section-hiking, and it was also convenient enough for Jeff and Heather to come and visit. They were two of our most ardent supporters, but they primarily supported us with prayer from their home because one month before we started the trail, Heather had given birth to their first child.

Because of their newborn they couldn't hike with us, but Heather said she had constantly prayed for us during early-morning feedings. It was nice to think that somebody else was awake, let alone praying for me, when I awoke each morning in the dark. They brought their baby boy with them that evening, and I got to carry him over the bridge that spans the Nolichucky on the outskirts of Erwin.

I should have been happy to see our friends; I should have been proud to make it to Erwin. I envisioned my entry into this hamlet in eastern Tennessee as a triumphant parade. But instead, I felt more like the fussy, red-faced baby I held in my arms.

Brew had been teasing me for the past several weeks, telling me that I had regressed to a toddler-like state on the trail. It was true. I existed on Juicy Juice mixed with water for my electrolyte drink, and I drank from a bottle with a nipple-shaped top. One of my special treats was chocolate milk, and like a two-year-old in diapers, I went through dozens of wet wipes every day. I had reached a point where I preferred mushy food to anything solid, and if I started crying it was usually because I needed food or wanted a nap.

Erwin was supposed to mark the conclusion of the almost-end and the beginning of the real-end. My increasing familiarity with the trail made the task seem that much harder. Suddenly it felt like every step I took pushed the finish line one step farther away. I thought about the never-ending climb up Big Bald that awaited me tomorrow, and I dreaded the unending PUDs between Camp Creek Bald and Hot Springs. I remembered how difficult the ascent up Snowbird Mountain was before entering Smoky Mountain National Park.

And then there was the park itself. At this point, I felt utterly weak with an eight-pound daypack resting on my shoulders. And in the Smokies I would have two thirty-mile stretches without a resupply. That meant more weight, slower miles, more calories burned, more calories *needed*, more sweating, more salt tablets, and more time away from Brew—the one person who could get me through anything.

I started to sniffle and tear up just like the two-month-old who was nestled against my sweaty synthetic T-shirt. Heather took her baby from me and then started soothing both of us.

"Jen, you are doing so great! You are only a week away from the finish. What's wrong?"

"I thought I would feel closer to the end in Erwin, and I don't," I said dejectedly. "A day out here feels like an eternity. A week is incomprehensible! I have given so much, and I feel so empty. I don't know if I have another seven days in me."

I realized that I seemed melodramatic, and I felt bad crying when I was so excited to see our friends. But the fact remained that even if I was able to keep hiking sixteen hours a day, I still had one-hundred and twelve hours to go and over three-hundred thirty miles of trail before reaching Springer Mountain. And that was still a really long way!

Heather stood next to me, patting my head, telling me how well I was doing, and mentioning several of the things I had to look forward to when I finished. Usually that was Brew's job. I looked around for my husband and saw him talking to Jeff near our friends' Subaru. In the twilight I could see his red, watery eyes, and I could tell Jeff was providing a pep talk similar to the one that Heather was giving me.

One of the reasons we decided to start the record attempt at Katahdin was to maximize daylight hours through Maine and New Hampshire and to get through the most technical portion of trail at the beginning. The other main reason was that we knew the closer we got to Springer Mountain, the more support we could receive from friends and family. It was a good strategy. We were both leaning harder and harder on the people who came to visit us, and we appreciated their support more and more.

Jeff and Heather provided us with compassion and words of encouragement, then they prayed with us. And before they left,

Heather brought out two trays of baked goods from her car and left them in our SUV. She also left us something even better—and there aren't many things I consider better than my friend's caramel brownies. But as Jeff and Heather turned on their headlights and pulled onto the two-lane road, Brew and I were not alone. Heather had left us her thirty-two-year-old marathon-running brother Hampton.

A few days ago Brew posed the question, "Do you think we would be in the same place on the trail if we had not asked so many people to come and help us?"

"I don't know," I replied. "Physically I've taken every step of this journey on my own, but emotionally I feel like our crew has carried me."

"Who do you think has been the most helpful crew member?"

"Well, Rambler was awesome, and he brought us Dutch, who was maybe the best hiker. We needed Warren for his wisdom up North and Melissa for her enthusiasm. And New York Steve and Horton were both a huge help in the mid-Atlantic. So . . . I don't know. They've all been valuable in different ways. It's been a combination of people and gifts that's allowed us to make it this far."

At that moment, I was eating a slice of supreme pizza that Brew had brought me from a nearby town.

"I guess our crew has been a little like this pizza," I said.

Brew asked me to explain.

"Well, you are the key ingredients—the crust and sauce and cheese. I know there's no way I could've ever made it here without you. You're irreplaceable, and you make this trip what it is, and our crew members are like the toppings. Some of them are like the protein because they provide physical strength; other people have been like vegetables that nurture me. But they all make it taste better."

"You sound hungry," said Brew. "I think you need to keep eating."

If our pit-crew was a pizza, then Hampton was the bacon because he added a lot of flavor.

Hampton was a runner and a triathlete. When he heard about our record attempt in the spring, he became immediately enthused and volunteered to help. Now that we were in Erwin, he had taken time off from his job to join us.

I adored hiking with Hampton. He constantly told me how great I was doing even when I was hiking uphill at a crawl. He filled the time by telling me about all the practical jokes that he had played on his friends—including putting a donkey in one of his buddy's basements and two turtles in a girlfriend's bathtub. With Hampton, I spent most of my time laughing and gasping. I told him that one of the most notorious tricks on the A.T. is to put a large rock in someone's pack when they're not looking. Then, knowing his mischievous nature, I warned him that if I found a rock in my daypack, I would punch him in the gut.

On a rainy evening, when we were hiking straight uphill toward Blackstaff Cliffs, Hampton and I had to focus more on our breathing than on our conversation. And after a particularly steep incline, we came to a place where the trail started to level out.

"You did it!" Hampton said. "You made it to the top. And let me just say, it was a treat watching your calf muscles on that last climb. I've never seen calf muscles like that on a girl!"

It was true. My calf muscles were scary-big. They were wider than my thigh with insane definition and a faint blue vein popping out in the middle. They could easily have given any Tour de France participant muscle envy (and that was without any EPO). However, my strong calves were also tired calves.

"Hampton, that was a false summit," I said. "We're not even halfway there yet."

"Oh," said Hampton. I was pretty sure I could feel his gaze return to my freakish leg muscles as we continued to climb.

Our uphill ascent was complicated by a steady rain. The path followed an old roadbed where off-road vehicles had left huge muddy ruts in the trail. As the rain intensified, the tread got softer. Now we were sliding out of our steps, losing ground and trying not to lose our shoes in the ankle-deep sludge.

I felt very present in that moment. My skin was wet, my legs were tired and covered in mud, my breathing was labored, and a thick veil of fog made it seem like we were gaining little ground on this sloppy ascent.

Then from behind me, Hampton asked, "So you wanna hear my version of the girl who got away?"

I looked back at him, a little surprised.

"You mean, relationship stories?"

"Yeah, relationships that I royally screwed up."

I *loved* hiking with Hampton. The next hour and a half was like listening to a sitcom. I heard about all the drama, all the mistakes, and all the awkward details that made me so glad I didn't have to date anymore.

We treaded lightly in the rain over the exposed rocks of Blackstaff Cliffs but instead of thinking about how one false step could end my record attempt, I listened to Hampton comically ramble on about bad timing, poor communication, and a lack of initiative. And despite his self-deprecating anecdotes, I made a mental list of all my girlfriends I could set him up with. Surely he had gotten it all out of his system by now. Right?

When we reached Hot Springs, we said good-bye to Hampton and hello to more friends who'd made the short trip from Asheville to cheer us on. I walked over the bridge that spans the French Broad River—the same river that comes within a mile of our front door in Asheville—listening to cheers and giving folks high fives.

Everything about this quasi-homecoming felt natural and wonderful, except when my friends tried to encourage me by telling me how close I was to the finish line.

We humans seem to struggle with ways to comfort one another in the face of adversity. I remember when Maureen found out that she had cancer. I told her, "Everything will be okay. You're one of the toughest women I know, so if anyone can defeat this illness, it's you." After my comment, I saw Maureen start to tear up and sit in silence.

I didn't realize until later how ignorant I'd been. Maureen had a progressive form of breast cancer. Things were *not* going to be okay—not for a long time. And I had just managed to make my good friend feel even worse.

Similarly, I did not want to hear from anyone else that I was "close to the finish." The people who were saying that were well meaning, but they hadn't thru-hiked the A.T. or a single forty-six-mile day in their entire lives. It didn't matter where I was located on the trail; every step was going to be hard until I reached Springer Mountain. It was only when I arrived at the end that things would finally be okay.

Past Hot Springs, I tried not to think about the remaining miles. Instead, I enjoyed a beautiful, quiet afternoon. I traveled through the dense hardwood forest, lost in thought and soaking in the peace and tranquillity of the woods.

The thin stretch of worn dirt that leads from downtown Hot Springs to the top of Snowbird Mountain is one of my favorite sections of the Appalachian Trail. The combination of shade and wind inside the rhododendron tunnels almost felt like an air conditioner—even on a late July afternoon. There is a hidden spring on this stretch, and I knew exactly where to find it. I dipped my bottle into the obscure pool and then brought it to my lips. The water tasted pure and sweet—better than anything that could ever come from a faucet.

I can always tell when I am getting close to Max Patch because I pass through a thick rhododendron tunnel that makes me feel like a gladiator walking through the underground passageways before entering the open air of the Colosseum. Max Patch is nature's arena. It is a wide grassy bald that sits close to the North Carolina-Tennessee border, and it provides 360-degree views of tall, rounded mountains with ever-changing shades of green, blue, and purple.

This mountain is where Brew and I shared one of our first dates. It's where I went with Maureen for a photo shoot a few months before she found out she was sick. It's also a place where I had many treasured memories from summiting the southern bald alone.

As I walked through the tall grass toward the summit, I saw Brew sitting at the top, waiting for me. He had hiked in a half mile, which was more ground than he was supposed to cover with his recovering ACL, but I didn't blame him for disregarding the doctor's orders. The healing properties of this bald outweighed the risk of injury.

We were fortunate enough to be the only two people there. When I reached the top, I rested for a few moments in my husband's arms. When we let go, I lifted my hands to the sky and let my hiking sticks dangle from the straps around my wrists. Then I turned in a slow circle to take it all in. The sun was kissing my face. The breeze was tickling my skin and filling my nostrils with the sweet scent of mountain air. It was a moment of dichotomy. I felt weak and strong, depleted yet filled, heavy but light, all at the same time.

Brew and I held hands as we walked side by side to the next road crossing.

"What are you thinking about?" asked Brew.

"Ancient Greek," I replied.

"Oh yeah?" asked Brew in a surprised tone.

"Mmm-hmm," I replied. "In my Greek class in college, we learned a lot of vocabulary. I've forgotten most of it, but one word that I still remember is *arete*. I guess it's really more of an esoteric concept than a vocab word."

"What does it mean?"

"From what I remember, it is the idea of reaching the fullest potential possible."

"So you think you are reaching your fullest potential on the trail?"

"Well, I hope so. I think so. But actually, I was thinking about *arete* on a bigger scale. Just now being on top of Max Patch with you, and walking down hand and hand, I sort of feel like life is at its fullest potential right now."

As I continued my walk that afternoon between Max Patch and Snowbird, it became clear to me that there was one other problem with friends telling me how close I was to the finish, another big reason why I didn't want to talk about the end of the hike; this was the only time in my entire life I could think of when I was giving all of myself to realize a dream.

Reaching for a life-long goal was rare enough, but actually being able to grab onto it seemed too good to be true. I was currently in a half-aware haze of turning my aspirations into a reality. It was a difficult and tangled but also beautiful and liberating place to be. And now I wondered, and even feared, what it would be like to wake up.

On the last mile leading to Snowbird Mountain, I hiked in the dusk longer than usual before pulling out my headlight. The sun had fallen from the sky, but my sense of the trail was so keen that I felt like I could anticipate the roots and rocks lining the path and could dance on top of them even in the dim twilight.

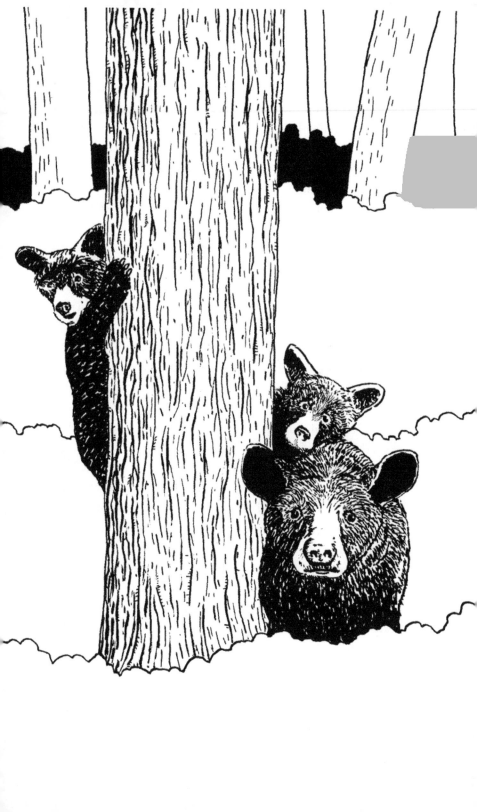

I was leaping from one obstacle to another when I heard a noise up ahead. Based on the volume and the type of rustling, I knew it was a bear. When I raised my chin, I saw not one but two cubs, and they were with their mother. Together, all three ran down the trail and around a turn to keep their distance. The problem was that I was headed in the same direction. As I neared the turn, I let out a loud cough. It worked. I heard the bears trample into the nearby forest.

I kept hiking without changing my pace. As soon as I rounded the bend, I looked downhill and saw one cub hugging the bark of a nearby oak tree, and the other peeking out from behind his mother. Even though she was within twenty yards, I didn't feel threatened.

I had seen lots of bears this summer—over thirty, in fact. Many of those sightings had been a mother with her cubs, and never once did a bear act aggressively. I also never felt as if the animals perceived me as a threat. I always tried to act natural, keep my distance, and maintain the same hiking pace. In doing that, it seemed that the bears viewed me and treated me like another wild animal. And that's exactly how I felt.

One aspect of the record attempt that I really loved was that I didn't have to leave the trail. The only times I did were to make a few late-night hotel runs. But even then, I always left in the dark and returned in the dark, so every waking hour for the past six weeks had been spent in the wilderness. I had never so fully immersed myself in nature. I had transitioned from a human seeking comfort to an animal migrating through the forest.

When I summited Snowbird, I could still make out the dark blue ridgeline of the Smoky Mountains as it contrasted against a deep gray sky. Brew and I shared another freeze-dried dinner and another night in our intimate two-person tent. I never reflected much before falling asleep on this trip—I was unconscious too quickly to do that. But as I settled into my sleeping bag that night, I was struck by the fact that more than forty days after we'd started, I was still doing what I loved, on a trail that I loved, with the man that I loved. And, yes, it was the hardest thing I'd ever done in my entire life. But it also felt like the best thing.

THE FINAL LEGS

JULY 27, 2011—JULY 31, 2011

When I arrived at the northern boundary of the Smoky Mountain National Park, I found Brew waiting there for me. It was still early in the morning, and our Highlander was the only car at Davenport Gap. I was in the middle of counting granola bars and energy chews for the next thirty-mile stretch, which I was planning to hike without support, when I heard a vehicle coming down the road. I looked behind me and saw a black-and-tan dog running beside the car. And the closer it came, the more familiar the dog looked.

Suddenly, I gasped, then yelled, "Uwharrie!"

Matt and Lily Kirk were inside the car, racing their four-legged family member up the road. I wasn't going to have to go through the Smokies alone!

I threw my arms around Brew's neck and kissed him.

"Thank you! Thank you, thank you, thank you! I can't believe you got Matt to come back!" I was like a kid who'd gotten just what she wanted from Santa. "This is *exactly* what I needed," I said.

Brew laughed as they climbed out of the car. "Don't thank me. Thank Matt and Lily. They're here because they wanted to come. Now go have some fun in the Smokies," Brew said, as he encouraged me toward the trail with a gentle pat on the butt. "I'll see you guys in thirty miles."

Matt had completed the section of Appalachian Trail through the Smokies eight times. And he arrived at the trailhead ready for his ninth adventure. After he told Lily and Uwharrie good-bye, we began the demanding ascent together.

Heading south into the Smokies from Davenport Gap, the trail gains 3,000 feet in the first five miles. Matt and I didn't talk much as I struggled to climb and eat my breakfast sandwich at the same time. Even when I was not eating, we did very little talking. We had caught up on conversation in Virginia, and now that we were in the Smokies, we were content to just hike.

The stretch of A.T. we were on felt like a combination treadmill and stair-stepper machine. Trail maintainers had placed logs across the path every few feet to guide water run-off, and their efforts created a very rhythmic hiking experience. One, two, three, four. One, two, three, four, and so on. The repetitive motion ushered my mind into a meditative trance, and before I knew it, we'd arrived on the ridge.

The crest of the Smokies is lined with evergreens. When the trees part, there are spectacular mountain views with the closer peaks appearing dark green and the distant ones fading into a light blue. The trail becomes very narrow in places, and the drop-off on either side can seem treacherous. A meticulous system of retaining walls that were built in the 1930's under FDR's New Deal keeps the trail intact and prevents washouts and rock slides. Even during the driest part of the summer, the trail here is lush. Everywhere you look, springs trickle out of the embankments and brightly colored moss borders the trail.

After hiking nearly sixteen miles, Matt and I were intercepted by a hiker from Knoxville who had walked up a side trail to replenish our food and supplies. He had emailed Brew several days before and offered to help us through the Smokies, so Brew had orchestrated a plan for him to meet Matt and me halfway through our section. It was a welcome surprise and an unexpected source of trail magic.

I was still in awe of the generosity that I received from people I knew and from people I had never met before. However, most of all, I was in awe of my husband. Brew never told me that new crew members were coming out until just before they arrived because he didn't want to get my hopes up and then have them not show. A few days earlier, I thought I would be traveling through the Smokies on my own with limited resupply. Now, thanks to my crew chief, I was able to enjoy seventy miles of companionship and an additional resupply.

Even though I was in the middle of a ten-hour stretch without seeing Brew, I was still well aware of his imprint on our trail adventure.

When I did finally get to see my husband at Newfound Gap, I noticed a positive change in his demeanor.

"You look different," I said.

"What do you mean?" he asked.

"I don't know. I guess you just look more relaxed than usual. What did you do today?"

"I drove down to Gatlinburg to get our car fixed. The mechanic got the window up, but the controls still don't work so I put some duct tape over them. Next, I got some groceries, then I washed our clothes at the Laundromat. But after that, I still had some time to kill, so I played eighteen holes of mini-golf."

My face lit up. My husband is at his absolute best when competing—even with himself. Mini-golf, bowling, batting cages, arcade games, board games, and recreational athletics all turn my husband into a kid at Disneyland. The knowledge that Brew had been able to enjoy himself, even for a few hours, made me really happy. It was the closest he had gotten to a vacation all summer.

That evening, Matt and I arrived at Clingman's Dome—the highest point on the entire trail—just after sundown.

We climbed silently to the observation tower on top of the mountain, and listened as our hiking poles clinked against the cement that led to the viewing area. When we made it to the top, we were the only people there. The sun had gone down, but we could still see the outline of the neighboring mountains. The valley floor was lighting up with street lamps and front-porch lights. It was as if the sky had inverted itself and all the stars had fallen to the ground. It was beautiful. It was worth the climb.

On day two in the park, Matt and I began hiking in the darkness and silence a little before five a.m. We traveled together on an overgrown trail through dew-soaked grass and copses of Frasier fir. Neither of us said a word for about two and a half hours, until I heard him stop behind me. "Look up," he said.

Thirty yards ahead, there was a black bear standing in the middle of the trail. He stared at us, and we stared back at him. Then, after several seconds, he finally moved a few steps farther down the trail. Matt and I took a few steps as well. The bear looked back at us, we looked at him, and once again he sauntered slowly along before stopping to see if we were still behind him.

The scenario repeated itself two or three more times, and in each instance, when the bear turned his head to look at us, he seemed more and more annoyed that we were still following him—not angry, just annoyed. He acted as if we had seriously inconvenienced him by disrupting his morning berries-and-bathroom routine. Like Matt and me, he was not quite ready for social interaction.

When the bear finally walked off the trail and Matt and I were able to pass, it was after eight a.m. and we were awake enough for conversation.

"Man, I'm glad the sun finally came up. I was tired of drooling on myself," said Matt.

I glanced back at him in confusion. I had no clue what he was talking about. Then I spotted the tiny LED light that was strung to a nearly invisible piece of thread around his neck. I wondered how he could use it without the elastic headband that secures it to the forehead. Then it came to me.

"You carry your headlamp in your mouth?!" I exclaimed.

Matt quickly defended himself. "Not having the elastic headband saves weight. And you don't *have* to wear your light on your head for it to be hands-free."

I loved the fact that Matt altered most of his gear and hiked in such a simple, Spartan style. But the image of him salivating on himself for the past two hours made me laugh so hard that I started to drool too.

That day, Brew had managed to break up our thirty-mile stretch by recruiting a friend from Asheville to hike in and meet us at Spence Field Shelter. Each extra resupply that Brew coordinated saved Matt and me from having to carry extra weight, and that resulted in extra energy. Extra energy meant stronger hiking, and

stronger hiking meant a faster time. We were still just a day ahead
of Andrew Thompson's record, so every minute mattered.

When Matt and I were running low on water, he was the one
who hiked off-trail to locate springs and refill our bottles. I was
able to stay put and eat, or keep hiking and wait for him to catch
up. But even with the added help, when we reached the turn-off
to Shuckstack Fire Tower and started the long, steep descent to
Fontana Lake, I felt weak and dizzy.

The switchbacks near the base of the mountain seemed never
ending. They reminded me of a dream I used to have about being
stuck in a stairwell that I couldn't escape. There were several places
where I thought I heard a road or believed I could see the blue
waters of Fontana, but by the time I reached the next switchback,
the noise or view had disappeared.

When Matt and I finally exited the woods at the base of the
Smokies to find our respective spouses, Uwharrie, and my dad
waiting for us, I almost couldn't believe they were real. But then
I sat down in our blue camp chair—the one that had cost us ten
dollars at a discount store—and nothing had ever felt so real, or so
comfortable. In fact, it felt like a throne. Over the past ten hours,
I had stopped for only a five-minute break at Spence Field Shelter.
We were now just one-hundred-fifty miles from the finish, and I
longed for the time when I could sit and rest for more than fifteen
minutes at a time.

On the banks of Fontana Lake, Matt and Lily bid us farewell,
but our number still stood at four. My dad had come to help us
finish, and somewhere near the next road crossing Maureen was
waiting to greet us with her tripod and camera. My father was the
one person who had greeted me at the end of the Appalachian
Trail in both 2005 and 2008, so now that he was here, the finish
felt more real.

I spent the next sixteen miles alone. For the first time on the
entire hike, I didn't just tell myself that I had what it took to set

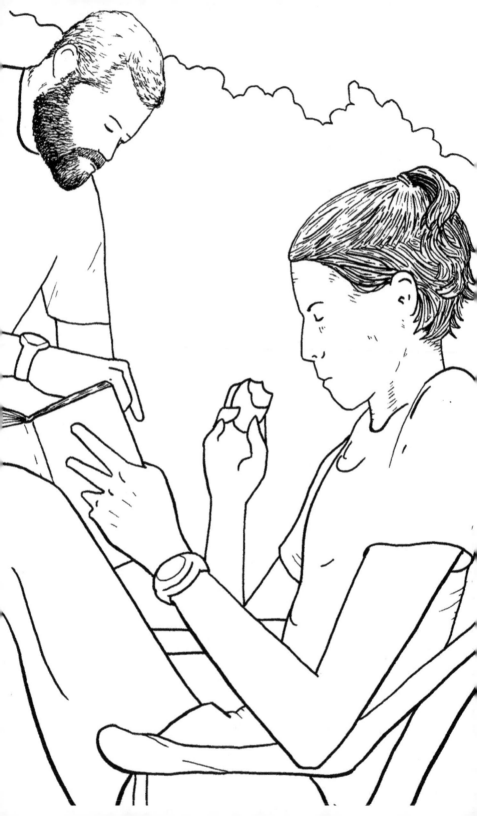

the record; I started to believe that I actually *would* set the record. I had reminded myself again and again on this journey that I belonged out here, but suddenly that statement no longer felt like self-affirmation. It felt like a fact.

When I arrived at Stecoah Gap, it was clear that while my anticipation and excitement had begun to increase, Brew was still business as usual. He did not talk about the finish or have a gleam in his eye that suggested we were close to the end. If anything, he seemed more uptight.

After a brief respite in Gatlinburg, it was now evident that Brew felt a huge amount of pressure to be perfect. We were potentially two and a half days away from Springer Mountain, and while that notion warmed my heart, it made my husband sick to his stomach.

His mind was traveling faster than I could hike. I could see the horrible hypothetical scenarios hidden in his tired eyes. If we did not succeed because of a missed road crossing or because he forgot to pack my EpiPen on a section where I got stung by bees, or if I should get sick from some piece of food that he handed me, then he would always feel as though he'd let me down. He never seemed to consider that he was the only reason I was in a position to be successful.

The next morning in the twilight, I hiked down from Cheoah Bald to the white rapids of the Nantahala River. Then I walked across the wooden bridge that carries the trail through the heart of the Nantahala Outdoor Center.

And as I began the calf-burning ascent out of the gorge—the most difficult climb that stood between me and Springer—I looked back and thanked Anne Riddle Lundblad for joining me.

Anne was voted the best female ultra-runner in North America in 2005 and 2006. She had won countless national and international races and was the silver medalist in 2005 at the USTAF 100k Championships in Japan. Even though Anne and I both lived in Asheville, I didn't know her that well. And that was my fault.

During our past interactions, she was always very kind and would ask thoughtful questions, and I would answer her with bright red cheeks, mumbling like I had pebbles in my mouth. And when she CC'ed me on a group email inviting me to train with her on the local trails, I was always too intimidated to respond because I felt like I was too slow.

Brew, however, had no problem communicating with Anne and asking her if she could help us this summer. And she eagerly agreed to come out for one of our final days.

Now, staring up at the steep ascent that led to Wesser Bald, I could think of no better hiking partner than Anne. I was too fatigued to act star struck, and I was immensely grateful to have such a talented athlete to help me.

Five minutes into my first two-sided conversation with Anne, I knew that I adored her. I asked her several questions about her most well-known athletic feats, and she indulged me with stories and answers. But in the end we spent most of our time talking about family, careers, books, and hobbies.

By the middle of the afternoon, my overall impression of Anne was that she was an amazing athlete, but that she was also extremely grounded. It was clear that the trail was not the most important thing in Anne's life, and I think that made her an even better runner. She didn't have to prove her identity in a race—that was already well established in the loving eyes of her daughter.

One thing I noticed when hiking with both Anne and Rebekah was that they seemed to be more well-rounded than the men I knew who had built comparable trail resumes.

"Do you think that being a woman helps you to be a better trail runner?" I asked.

"What do you mean?" Anne replied.

"Well, I was just thinking about it, and it seems to me like Mother Nature forces us to take breaks. Whether it is a monthly break for our cycle, or a seasonal one to have children, we're not always expected to perform at our best. It's like we have an excuse— a damn good excuse—to take breaks. I almost feel bad for men who have the pressure of competing at a high level *all* the time."

"I hadn't thought about it that way," said Anne. "But I know that without breaks, I probably would have burned out by now."

"You know, it might seem crazy, but sometimes I think we have a leg up when it comes to endurance sports," I suggested. "After all, women outlive men, and we're also the ones who give birth. So when it comes to longevity and pain, it seems like we might have an evolutionary advantage."

Anne laughed and said, "I like that theory."

All day Anne and I talked and hiked, and the miles seemed to fly by without either of us much noticing. I was surprised when we left Highway 64 and the sun started to go down. The day had passed quickly, and now I found myself night-hiking for what I hoped would be the second-to-last time on this trip. Anne and I walked in the dark with our headlamps on toward the fire tower that crowned Albert Mountain.

"I've been meaning to thank you for giving a presentation at my daughter's school last year," said Anne.

"It was fun," I responded. "I love talking about the A.T. and getting kids excited about the trails and the outdoors."

"Well, my daughter was definitely inspired."

"Really?" I asked.

"Yeah, she thinks you are a rock star, which is funny considering she simply tolerates most of my races."

"Do you want her to be a runner?" I asked.

"No," said Anne. "Not unless she wants to be. I just want her to find something she loves and be able to pursue it."

All of a sudden the lack of calories and sleep deprivation

brought to light what I had been trying to make sense of for so many miles.

Multiple people had told me that I was a role model for going after this record. And that hadn't really made sense to me. After all, this type of endeavor probably appeals to less than 0.01% of the people out there. I mean, how does hiking the Appalachian Trail in a short amount of time positively impact anyone? But Anne made me realize that being a role model isn't about inspiring other people to be like *you*; it is about helping them to be the fullest version of *themselves*.

The main legacy of this endeavor would not be to encourage others to set a record on the Appalachian Trail, but to encourage them to be the best form of their truest selves. And it just so happened that my best form was a hiker.

When I went to bed that evening, it was with the knowledge that the next day, I would walk into Georgia. I had roughly ninety-five miles to go and just one more full day and night on the trail, so I wanted to make the most of it.

"Are you really setting your alarm for 2:45 a.m.?" asked Brew.

"Yep."

"But it's already past eleven," he protested.

"I know."

"Do you think it's safe to be this tired already and hike for five hours in the dark on so little sleep?"

"I think the safest thing to do is to try to finish as quickly as possible," I said. "The longer I am out here, the more potential there is for error."

Brew shrugged.

"Well, at least you'll be hiking with Carl. Make sure you go slow, okay?"

"Okay," I promised. Then instead of saying good night, I looked at my husband and said, "Good nap."

Brew chuckled. "Yeah, 'good nap' to you, too."

Roughly three hours later, I woke up. After gagging on a protein shake and energy bar inside the tent, I crawled out to find myself in the middle of Carl's headlamp beam. I am sure I was not a pretty sight.

I'd never met Carl before 10:45 the previous night, when he had arrived at our campsite just as Anne left. He was a friend of Matt Kirk's, and he lived and trained in the North Georgia mountains. He'd agreed to hike with me the last day and a half—when I was at my most delirious—to ensure that I didn't wander off-trail or, God forbid, start hiking north by accident.

I half groaned and half growled at Carl to acknowledge his presence. Together we located the trail, and for the next five hours, I centered my headlight on his large gray sneakers, never once averting my gaze. However, I did remember views from this section, so when we passed a rock outcropping on our left, I could imagine the dark valley below us. And when we arrived at the sign pointing toward Carter Gap Shelter, I pictured the original, primitive lean-to built by the Civilian Conservation Corps and the more modern structure nearby with additional sleeping space and a covered porch.

You'd think I'd have built up some confidence after covering 2,100 miles in forty-five days, but I was still in awe of, if not flat-out intimidated by, the athletic caliber of our support crew. Carl was no exception. Then again, he would have intimidated most people. He was hardcore.

For one thing, he looked hardcore. He was several inches taller than I was, but unlike Dutch or Matt, who looked down at me but probably weighed less than I did, Carl was a tank. He looked more like a lumberjack than an ultra-runner. He had thick, muscular legs and broad, defined shoulders.

Carl did things that were hardcore, too. He didn't bother with ordinary ultra-races; instead he only signed up for the most sadistic races in the country, the ones put on by Gary Cantrell.

The most notorious of these races was the one-hundred-mile Barkley Marathon. The route had nearly 60,000 feet of elevation gain and another 60,000 of loss. It had been going on for twenty-five years, yet it had only thirteen finishers. Andrew Thompson was one. So was David Horton. Carl was not a finisher yet, but he probably would be soon. There were no female finishers—but I couldn't think about that, not right now, at least.

At that moment, what Carl and I were doing did not even remotely compare to the Barkley. All we had to do was hike sixty miles to Tesnatee Gap.

In a way, sixty miles should not have seemed that far. I had strung together several back-to-back fifty-mile days already. And the thought of being close to the end should have carried me down the trail effortlessly. The problem was that the idea of the finish remained in my head and had not yet infused my body with extra energy.

The idea of putting my body through another sixty-mile day, at the end of a 2,100 mile journey, seemed unbearable if not impossible. I had started this hike with a full tank of energy and athleticism. Now my energy gauge was on empty—even the fumes had dissipated.

It was hard to drink, hard to eat, it was even hard to form words to communicate my thoughts. Every step and every breath was labored. So far, my mind and body had worked in tandem, propelling me down the trail each day. But at this point, there was a strong disconnect between what my mind wanted and what my body could do. I started praying my way down the trail; begging

God to give me a little bit more energy and enough strength to reach the finish.

Carl, on the other hand, was fresh, and he was only out here for a day and a half. After finishing nearly eighty miles at the Barkley, surely he could do sixty miles in the mountains of north Georgia. Right?

But while it was true that my new hiking partner was not as worn down as I was, it turned out he was suffering from one of the most notorious and debilitating organisms found on the trail. Carl was carrying a protozoan parasite in his digestive tract called giardia.

Giardia makes you feel like someone is constantly punching you in the stomach. It causes explosive, unrelenting diarrhea, which quickly leads to dehydration. Even after you survive the initial symptoms, you will feel completely depleted and more than a little worried every time you need to pass gas. Carl had contracted giardia a month ago by drinking untreated water from an impure source, and he was still suffering from some of the unpleasant side effects. His frequent side trips off the trail reminded me of how miserable I'd felt in Vermont when I fell victim to similar symptoms.

You would think that seeing our able-bodied crew at the next road crossing would have been uplifting, but they were as motley and as haggard as we were. Brew was there rummaging around our disorganized car with a big black brace on his right knee. But the four-inch scar from his ACL surgery didn't look half as gnarly as the back of his left leg. He had come in contact with some poison ivy near the Nantahala Outdoor Center, and now he had a dime-sized, puss-filled blister surrounded by pink welts that seemed to spread by the minute.

Next to Brew stood Maureen. Finished with her initial treatments and not yet in remission, Maureen was yelling at Brew for letting the SUV that she had cleaned just ten days ago regress back into a disheveled mess of granola bars, damp worn socks, camping equipment, and first-aid supplies—all speckled white from a Gold Bond powder explosion.

On top of that, my dad had gone missing. Apparently, he was roaming around Hiwassee, Georgia, running errands and trying to buy my husband a new phone. For the second day in a row, Brew had managed to sabotage a cell phone—this time by dropping it in a Dairy Queen Blizzard. Now my sweet father was trying to buy my husband a new one while also assuming the role of central command since *his* phone actually worked.

Even our car was showing signs of wear and tear. It had a red, muddy bottom and a dry, dusty top. Brew had refused to wash it since leaving Maine because he thought the dirt and filth brought us good luck. And it didn't really make sense to clean the outside of the car when we were still putting our soiled and smelly clothes, gear, and bodies on the inside. We'd taped artwork from our goddaughter and neighbors and well-wishes from our cousins to the ceiling above the passenger seat. And we'd covered the buttons on the driver's-side door with duct tape to prevent us from accidentally rolling down the window when we couldn't get it up again.

There we all sat at a road crossing near Hiwassee, Georgia, in hundred degree heat on July 30. I was a zombie, Carl had diarrhea, Brew had the beginning stages of a staph infection behind his left knee, Maureen had cancer, my dad was MIA, and our car had entirely lost its resale value. As a team, we didn't look like we could win a 5k, let alone set a record on the Appalachian Trail. But this trip had taught me that a trail record wasn't about looking good; it was all about survival.

Sensing the despair of our ragtag team, Carl spoke up. "This is what it's *supposed* to feel like," he said.

I was too tired to ask what he meant, but I was pretty sure that I agreed with his comment. I'd dealt with discomfort and pain this entire summer, but I'd continually told myself that the negative side effects of hiking forty-seven miles a day for forty-six days were perfectly normal.

I assumed that these effects were both understudied and unknown. I told myself that shin splints and stomach bugs were standard, that nausea was normal, and that exhaustion was expected.

Carl was right. After what we had all been through—independently and collectively—I don't think we could have felt any other way.

That afternoon, the humidity and heat were oppressive. The ground was parched, and chalky red dust kicked up every time I took a step. On the last full day of the women's record hike, the conditions had been identical, and I had come as close as I ever had to stepping on the head of a rattlesnake who was sunning himself on the trail. The vivid memory caused me to pay close attention to where I placed my feet. And yet, I *still* almost repeated my 2008 rattlesnake encounter when I stepped within striking distance of a snake sunning itself near the trail. In addition to my snake run-in, the crew had seen a black bear at one of the road crossings, and Brew was dive-bombed by a screech owl on a side trail as he tried to bring me a milkshake. The adventure was nearing its end, but that didn't mean an end to the adventure.

When we reached Unicoi Gap, it was already six p.m. and I still had fourteen miles to cover. Carl agreed to walk with me for the last stretch, and his company was invaluable. We made it up the steep climb to Blue Mountain Shelter and across the rock fields near Chattahoochee Gap to reach the old railroad bed before dark. I loved it when the trail followed old logging roads and railroad beds. The width of the trail increased, there were fewer roots and rocks, and the grade was far gentler than most other stretches. Now, more than ever, I appreciated the gradual incline and lack of debris on the three-mile section into Low Gap Shelter. But soon after, the path left the worn trading route and returned to the natural contours of the forest. It was dark, I was following Carl's shoes once again, and the trail kept going uphill.

I continued to hike, but started to feel claustrophobic with the dark closing in around me. I suddenly struggled to breathe, and more than that, my heart started to hurt. I had felt slight pains in my chest during the past two weeks, but I didn't want to tell Brew about them because they were relatively minor and I didn't want him to worry. But this time, it felt like my heart was cramping instead of beating, and my chest felt like it had a cinder block on top of it. The dull pain ached in my core.

I struggled to take a few more steps, then I fell to the trail, gasping for breath. I was hyperventilating, and my eyes started to water. Carl rushed to my side and asked if I was okay. I nodded yes, but then I continued to wheeze as tears streamed down my face.

I tried to relax and control my breathing as Carl sat behind me and massaged my shoulders.

"It'll be okay," he said. "Just focus on your breathing. In through your nose, out through your mouth."

His response was perfect. Even in the moment, I thought how nice it was to have someone as hardcore as Carl rubbing my back and soothing me with his words. His sympathy and the fact that he didn't freak out—at least visibly—helped put me at ease.

When my breathing slowed down, Carl reached into his daypack and offered me food and water. I sat there sniffling, breathing, and shoving energy chews into my mouth until I started to feel better.

Finally, I felt good enough to stand and keep hiking. Carl continued trying to take my mind and his off my sudden chest constrictions, the consuming darkness, and the steep ascent that taunted us with every step.

"Hey, isn't that Mumford and Sons song that Brew played at one of the road crossings, like, your theme song for the summer?" he asked.

I nodded my head, still a little winded.

"I have it on my iPhone if you want to hear it."

My typical view of cell phones on the trail was that they were for emergency use only, but this still felt like an emergency to me.

"Yeah, that would be nice," I replied.

So, hiking on a ridge in north Georgia, in a darkness so thick that it made me lose track of time and space, Carl and I listened to "The Cave."

I had heard the song several dozen times over the past few weeks. The beat was catchy, the lyrics were poetic; it just resonated with me on multiple levels. But so far, I hadn't taken the time to figure out why.

On this dark, warm night in the heart of backcountry Georgia, the song's relevance to my situation became painfully clear. I listened to the verses as if for the first time. They called to me as if speaking in tongues only I could understand.

"It's empty in the valley of your heart.
The sun, it rises slowly as you walk
Away from all the fears,
And all the faults you've left behind."
• • •
"Cause I have other things to fill my time.
You take what is yours and I'll take mine.
Now let me at the truth,
Which will refresh my broken mind."

Immediately, I flashed back to the Long Trail, when I was hiking away from my brokenness. Everything seemed wrong. My life seemed shattered. Yet I managed to keep moving forward, and move away from the pain, toward love.

"So tie me to a post and block my ears.
I can see widows and orphans through my tears.
I know my call despite my faults,
And despite my growing fears."

This verse alluded to Odysseus, my trail name's namesake. He tied himself to the ship's mast and filled his crew's ears with wax to block out the Sirens' song. Likewise, we took great measures to stay on course and limit our distractions. I was out here for a reason. I believed in my heart that the trail was a *calling*. And yes, there was suffering—both on the trail and off. The pain was hard and real. But at the end of the day, I had a choice to hide from it or hike through it.

"So come out of your cave walking on your hands,
And see the world hanging upside down.
You can understand dependence
When you know the maker's land."

Like Plato's cave dweller, I had been exposed to a new reality on the trail. It was my job to explore it even if I didn't fully understand it. But I needed help—dependence was imperative. At no other time in my life had I felt more reliant on my faith, my husband, and the people who surrounded us, or on the living spirit of the earth, than on this journey. And only in being completely dependent did I feel strong and free.

Finally, the chorus sounded one last time:

"And I will hold on hope
And I won't let you choke

On the noose around your neck
And I'll find strength in pain
And I will change my ways
I'll know my name as it's called again."

This song, this hike, this whole experience, that started from the day I left Springer Mountain as a twenty-one-year-old was all about hope. I knew about the darkness—the hanging I'd encountered on my first hike and the abduction of Meredith three years later. I had faced deaths, doubts, and fears. But the trail had provided a way to move past those obstacles and keep hiking forward. The forest had allowed me to find my true self. I had heard my name as it was called. And I'd become Odyssa.

The song ended. Carl turned off his iPhone and put it back in his daypack.

"You know, that's not really a fun song," he said.

"I know," I replied. "It's better than fun."

We kept hiking for what seemed like forever, hoping that each new turn would bring us to the next road. Finally, before we knew how close we were, we heard a cry in the darkness.

"Sixty *freak-ing* miles!"

Brew had spotted our headlamps bobbing through the forest, and his voice let us know that we were within fifty yards of the Gap. We'd made it. This was our last night on the trail.

I lay down on my foam sleeping pad at 11:30 that evening, and once again set my alarm for 2:45 a.m. Brew didn't fight me this time; we both wanted to be done.

Then, as I wrapped a sleeping-bag liner around my torso, I felt another twinge in my heart. In a strange way, I was glad that it hurt. Well, maybe I wasn't glad. But it just felt right, like it *should* hurt. Because sometimes things have to hurt before they can grow. And because of this adventure, my heart felt larger, stronger, and more full.

When I awoke on the last morning of the hike, I felt more miserable than excited. Every part of me hurt, and every part was exhausted.

I got dressed, crawled out of the tent, and began trudging along behind Carl's feet. I purposefully tried not to engage with him. I didn't even want to fully open my eyes. The closer I could come to sleep-walking, I thought, the better.

It was still pitch-black when we made it to Neels Gap. Brew had set up two chairs by the car, and he handed us both a hard-boiled egg tortilla wrap. I had eaten many of these protein-packed wraps on the trail. Sometimes Brew added cheese, but mostly it was just two eggs and some salt in a flour tortilla. But this time, as soon as I put the wrap near my mouth, I started to gag. Then Carl saw me out of his peripheral vision and instinctively began dry heaving too.

"I can't stay here," I said. "I'll eat something on the trail. I really don't want to throw up."

I stood up and Carl followed. He stuffed several granola bars and two full water bottles in his waist pack and we were off.

However, before we even made it to the trailhead across the road, Carl had to stop and bend over. His whole body was convulsing in more dry heaves—and I could feel the bile building up in my throat.

"Carl, I have to keep going," I said. "If I see *you* puke, *I'm* going to puke."

Carl nodded his head, and I was off.

By the time I made it to the summit of Blood Mountain at the first light of day, I expected to hear Carl hiking up behind me. I called out his name, but there was no response. I kept hiking but walked slower. He had all our food and liquids and I really needed a pick-me-up. I had barely eaten at the campsite that morning because I knew I would see Brew in less than five miles. But at Neels Gap, I was too nauseous to eat. Now, I was on the southern slope of Blood Mountain, and my stomach was *screaming* for food. I'd hiked sixty miles yesterday and had come over 2,150 miles in the last month and a half. All that my body wanted to do was eat, and I didn't have any food to give it.

Being famished and light-headed would not have worried me as much except that the last two times I'd felt this way, I'd passed out.

Once after an Ironman triathlon and another time while hiking the Pacific Crest Trail, I had similar feelings of dizziness and low blood sugar. In both instances, I woke up on my back without remembering how I'd gotten there.

All summer, I had been very careful to monitor my caloric intake and carry a few snacks, even if a friend was muling me. But now on the last day, my fatigue and laziness had caused me to make a poor decision, and I was afraid I would pay for it by losing consciousness.

I had come all this way, and now there was a possibility that I would have a medical emergency and ruin my chance of setting the record with less than twenty-six miles to go.

I decided to sit down, figuring I wouldn't fall as far if I fainted, and that I could rest while I waited for Carl to catch up.

I sat in the middle of the trail, calling for him every few minutes. I was probably there for twenty or thirty minutes, but it was long enough to realize that Carl was not coming. I kept thinking, *He should be here by now. Something must be wrong.*

My personal fear turned into worry for Carl. Was he okay? Should I go back and look for him? I didn't know what to do.

Finally, I decided that I didn't know where Carl was or how to find him, but I did know that I had six miles to the next road, and I should do everything in my power to make it there safely.

I stood up and started to hike. Surprisingly, instead of feeling depleted, I felt like I was floating. It was a weird, almost out-of-body experience. I was breathing through my nose, my mind felt disconnected from my feet, and I was flying down the trail. I remember Matt Kirk sharing a story about being in dire need of food and reaching a transcendent state of gliding down the trail— followed by several intense hallucinations.

This must have been the feeling he was describing. Fortunately, I wasn't hallucinating yet. At least I didn't think I was.

When I was two miles from the road crossing, I heard a noise I didn't recognize. It was very loud, almost as if there were a storm or groundswell coming from the forest floor. I kept floating along and staring into the woods, when suddenly I saw two large wild boars. They saw me, too, and ran, crashing through the underbrush. But instead of charging farther away, they ran straight across the trail—fifteen yards ahead of me.

I was stunned to see the two portly animals with short, stiff legs move so quickly. And I was even more surprised to see the two adults followed by a dozen or so farrows, or baby boars. They were a collage of colors: pink, brown, gray, and black. Before this encounter, I had only seen four boars in all my years of hiking in the Appalachian Mountains. And now I was convinced that there was a polychrome family of fourteen running out of sight.

When I got to the next road crossing, Brew looked shocked to see me exit without Carl.

"What happened? Where's Carl?" he asked.

"I don't know," I said. "I hoped he would be with you. I never even saw him. I thought he bailed before Blood Mountain and went back to Neels Gap. All I know is that I just encountered a whole lot of animals and I'm not sure they were all real. I need some food, and I need it *now*."

I sat down and started chugging a Coca-Cola. The sugar revived me like an IV pumping through my veins. Next, I began to work on the hard-boiled burrito that Brew had made earlier. Three hours ago it had made me retch. Now it smelled tempting and tasted delicious.

As I started to feel better, I also started to get excited. I looked around and saw James and my oldest brother, Jones, standing by the car and pulling out gear so they could hike the last twenty miles with me. Maureen was there smiling and taking even more photos than usual.

I felt warm and full inside. It was probably a result of the egg burrito and the Coke, but there was also a part of me that felt satisfied by more than just food.

I glanced over at Brew, who was calling Carl from a borrowed cell phone while simultaneously rummaging through the trunk of our car to pick out my snacks and refill my water bottles.

"There's no answer," Brew said with a concerned and frustrated look on his face.

I told my husband the same thing I had repeated in my head for the past six miles. I said, "Carl will be fine. He is an experienced runner, and he knows these woods like the back of his hand. He can take care of himself."

"I hope so," responded Brew.

Then I asked, "Honey, do you *feel* it at all?"

"Feel what?" he replied.

"The finish."

"We're still twenty miles from Springer Mountain," said Brew matter-of-factly. "When you hike another nineteen miles and when we find Carl, *then* it will feel like the finish."

I knew that my husband was not trying to be a killjoy. He

was just staying focused. And I needed to stay focused as well. I couldn't let go of my emotions or my intensity just yet. But repressing my joy was a lot harder with my oldest brother standing five feet from me.

Jones had never come to the trail before. He had a frenetic, high-powered banking job that made it difficult for him to take time off. The fact that he was here, in the middle of nowhere Georgia, where his Blackberry didn't work, helped me to realize just how special and important this day was going to be.

He and I set out together to hike the next section while James and Brew stayed at Woody Gap to wait for Carl.

It proved to be an exceptionally entertaining stretch, especially since we didn't hike. In fact, it was the first time all summer that I ran for an extended period of time. I'd started out from Woody Gap with a brisk hiking pace, but my brother was soon goading me from behind. "This is runnable. Why aren't you running this?"

"Jones," I replied in a mixture of consternation and amusement, "I haven't run all summer."

To which he responded, "Well, better late than never. C'mon, pick up the pace!"

The prodding was so good-natured and humorous that I decided to appease him. I could hear Brew's voice in the back of my head, saying, "Slow down. It is not worth it to run on your very last day and risk an injury." But I couldn't help it. All summer long, ultra-runners, endurance junkies, even a national magazine writer had tried to get me to transition from walking my miles to running them. Yet the only person who succeeded at the task was my brother, who spent eighty hours a week in a cubicle in Manhattan.

As we trotted down the trail, Jones kept provoking me over and over. But beyond reminding me to keep my cadence up, he also kept saying things like, "It's so beautiful out here," and "All you have to worry about is food and water. This is the life!"

My brother was right. Compared to his high-tech, high-speed world, my existence for the past forty-six days had been wonderfully simple. I had spent the summer going three miles per hour, never once having to look at a computer or use my phone except in emergencies. It's amazing that even setting a speed record on the Appalachian Trail seemed unhurried when compared to our modern existence.

When Jones and I jogged out of the woods at our next road crossing, Brew's jaw dropped.

"What are you doing?" he asked.

"My brother the banker wouldn't let me walk," I replied.

Brew laughed and shook his head. "Just be careful," he warned. "Really, *really* careful."

"I will, I promise. Have you heard from Carl?"

"Yeah, he tried to catch up with you, but kept getting sick," Brew said. "He ended up taking a side trail to a nearby road. I think your dad's on his way to pick him up."

I gladly let go of the notion that some grave misfortune might transpire in the eleventh hour. Now that Carl was accounted for, there was nothing keeping us from Springer Mountain.

After a quick snack, I returned to the woods with my other brother, James.

"Don't you think this is runnable?" he asked.

I looked back in disbelief, only to see him chuckling.

My brothers like to claim that they were the ones responsible for making me tough and determined. However, if anyone was responsible for making me—and my brothers—that way, it was my mother. All three of us had grown up hearing the same phrases over and over again. My mom was like a broken record when we were upset, always repeating lines like, "Life's not fair" or "Oh, get over it—you're fine." When my brothers picked on me, she would say, "Don't give them an emotional payoff." And the phrase I heard most often was, "Quit being such a drama queen!"

Often, I was envious of my friends, whose mothers coddled them, but I was now convinced more than ever that God knew exactly what he was doing when he assembled our family. I might not have always received the empathy that I wanted, but I had the mom, dad, and brothers that I needed.

When I arrived at Three Forks, Brew was there, and not far away was a man with a cap, white beard, and round belly who was standing in a creek. As I drew closer, I could tell that the man in the water was Warren. Before Brew could say a word, Warren started calling out to me like a preacher from a pulpit.

"From the currents of Katahdin Stream, you have traveled along the worn peaks of the mighty Appalachian Mountains—mountains formed by the rivers and worn by the rain. Now here you stand, at the base of Springer Mountain, and it is time to drink once again."

Warren reached down into the water and filled his dented metal cup. Then he handed it to me. The man who'd never once tasted bottled water was offering me a sip of refreshment from the only catchment device he ever carried on the trail.

I brought the cup to my lips and drank. Warren grinned.

I wiped the extra water from my lips with the back of my wrist and handed the cup back to him. "Thank you," I said.

Then I sat down to eat some potato chips while Warren remained in the water, dividing the currents with his strong, thick calves. The front of his green shirt had a white blaze printed on it, the ubiquitous sign of the Appalachian Trail. He stood so still and silent that it almost looked like he was an actual trail marker. And for me, at least, I think he was.

It was strange to see Warren again, now that I was so close to the end. He had been there before I began my first A.T. journey. He had helped me plan for the Long Trail. He was a constant friend and mentor. But the last time I saw him in Vermont, he was also a source of frustration.

Warren had known all too well the obstacles that awaited me. He painted too realistic a picture of what I would have to endure to be successful. But at the base of Springer Mountain, there was no one I would have rather had with me.

Of all the people who would surround me on top of Springer, only Warren could truly empathize with what my body and mind had been through over the last month and a half. And he was one of the few people who could ever fully appreciate what we had accomplished.

As I continued to shove Kettle chips into my mouth, Brew asked, "Do you want to change out any gear for the last section?" He froze for a moment and said, "Wow. Did I really just say 'the last section'?" Then he immediately returned his attention to my daypack.

This was our final road crossing before the Springer Mountain parking lot, and while I'd had some time over the past few hours to wrap my head around the end, it was clear that Brew still couldn't comprehend the words coming out of his own mouth. Even though he had said "the last section," he didn't once mention the finish, the record, or the people who would be waiting for us on top of the mountain. He was entirely focused on whether I had the right food and enough water. He checked to make sure I had Benadryl and an EpiPen, and then he looked at the map to make sure he could navigate the maze of dirt roads.

As I put the potato chips down and stood up, Brew held out my daypack. I took it from him, then held on to his hand and gave it a squeeze. Then I let go and turned to see James waiting by the trailhead. I walked over to join my brother, and together we disappeared into the woods. It was the last section of the entire trail, and all I had to do to reach my goal was hike to Brew.

As we climbed toward the Springer Mountain parking lot, James and I were both pretty quiet. I'm not sure if we didn't know what to say or if there just weren't words to express how we felt. Every now and then, I would childishly blurt out, "Oh my gosh . . . oh my gosh . . . oh my gosh." But then I would revert to a far more expressive silence.

· 15 ·

THE RECEPTION

JULY 31, 2011

When we arrived at the Springer Mountain parking lot, the small gravel clearing was packed full of cars, more than I had ever seen there. And in contrast to the array of cars in the parking lot, I could see only two people standing there. A few yards away, surrounded by SUVs, stood Brew. He had his arms crossed and he was wearing a crooked smile. Tears were welling up in his eyes. For the first time in forty-six days, his posture and the look on his face seemed relaxed, almost limp. The burden he had put on himself—the burden not to let me down—had finally been lifted. The tunnel vision he'd had for so long seemed to have faded, and in its place had emerged a new expression.

When people ask me why I would want to set the record, or what I could possibly gain from hiking the trail in forty-six days, I think back to the contented look I shared with Brew in the Springer Mountain parking lot. That one glance made every step, every mountain, every ailment, every storm, every discomfort, and every tear worthwhile. No trophy or winner's purse could ever match the value of looking into the eyes of my husband, knowing that together we had accomplished the impossible.

Brew and I walked toward each other and wrapped ourselves in a teary, tight embrace.

"You did it," he whispered.

"No, *we* did it," I replied.

We hugged and cried for a long moment, and then Brew pulled away and reached for my hand. It was time.

We had one more mile to hike to reach the southern terminus of the Appalachian Trail, and we were going to walk every step hand in hand.

Looking toward the trailhead that led up Springer, I smiled at the only other person in the parking lot. Squatting by the path, waiting for us to hike toward her, was my mother. She was kneeling down to take photos of us as we began the final mile of our journey. Having my mom there made a perfect moment even better. We had both come such a long way.

The walk to the top of Springer was filled with silence. I alternated between taking deep breaths and choking up on tears and emotions. Brew gingerly walked by my side, watching his foot placement to avoid reinjuring his ACL. This was farther than he'd hiked all summer. My mother and brother followed a few dozen yards behind.

At one point, Brew asked, "Do you want me to tell you who is waiting at the finish?"

I shook my head. I wanted it to be a surprise.

Brew then asked, "Do you want to hug any of your friends before you touch the rock?"

I looked at him like he was crazy.

"First we touch the rock," I said. "*Then* we visit."

"Okay, okay," he said with a quiet laugh. "That's why I'm asking."

When we came within a few hundred yards of the summit, we saw a collage of bright colors through the trees. We entered the clearing that marks the top of Springer Mountain. The exposed granite leading to the plaque that marks the southern terminus was hidden by a group of people. I heard the cheering and noticed the crowd, but I maintained my focus and walked straight to the boulder that bears the worn bronze sign that signifies the southern terminus of the Appalachian Trail.

Together, Brew and I placed our hands on it. Then we embraced each other once again. I looked at the watch on my wrist, which was draped around my husband's neck. Through smiles and sobs, I did the math. Forty-six days, eleven hours, and twenty minutes after I left Katahdin, we had reached Springer Mountain. Now *that* was a positive number.

We had beaten the previous record by twenty-six hours. I couldn't decide if twenty-six hours seemed like a fleeting moment or an eternity. I guess in the end it didn't matter. I had done my absolute best and I could walk off this mountain never wondering what might have been.

My tears increased as I sat down beside my husband and buried my head in his seven-week beard. They weren't sad tears—not entirely—nor did they flow from joy or exhaustion. I think they were "everything" tears. For the past month and a half I had suppressed all of my feelings—pain, happiness, fear, disappointment, excitement, anticipation, and every other emotion that might

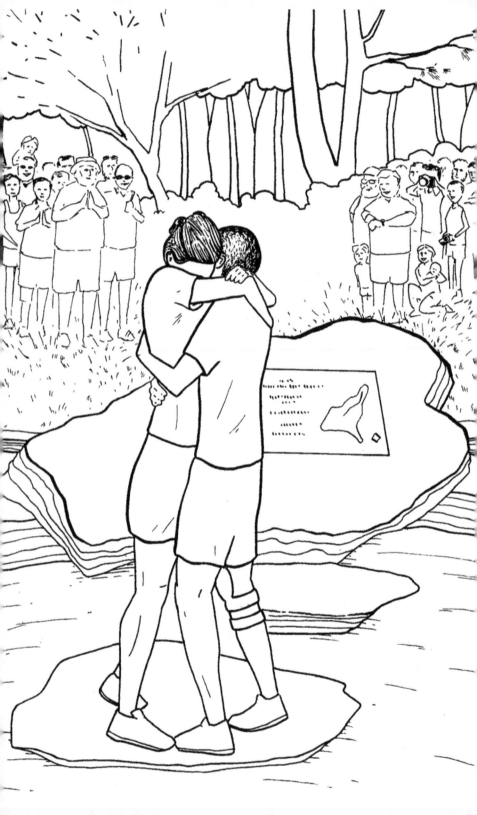

have threatened to take my mind off the ultimate goal. Now I could finally let them out. Unfortunately, the emotional cocktail created a confused, blotchy, tear-streaked expression on my face. There would be no glamour shots at *this* finish line.

Brew and I stood there and cried for what was probably an awkwardly long amount of time for our bystanders. Eventually, I rubbed my eyes and started to look around and make out individuals in the crowd, one by one. I saw my college roommate, my pen pal from summer camp, our neighbors from home, my in-laws. There were dogs, digital cameras, and babies—lots of babies. I was amazed that so many of our friends had brought their infants and toddlers to the top of Springer in ninety-degree heat. Trail friends were there—including Warren, who stood off in the distance to take it all in. And there were a few faces that I didn't recognize. But out of the fifty or so people on top of the mountain, almost everyone had come because they were somehow interwoven into our lives.

Looking out at the crowd, it almost felt as if Brew and I were back at our wedding weekend. The people who meant the most to us were all there. There were pictures being taken and congratulatory hugs being exchanged. Our friend Alice even uncorked a bottle of champagne that she'd carried in her purse.

The scene—and probably the champagne, since it was the first sip of alcohol I had consumed in a month and a half—caused me to reminisce about our wedding ceremony. The event that had taken place in Virginia three summers ago had been beautiful and memorable. But I think I preferred the occasion we shared on top of Springer Mountain even more.

There was no pomp and circumstance. I wasn't wearing a beautiful dress, and Brew and I did not exchange traditional vows. Instead, we professed our love through the actions of the past forty-six days. The trail had brought to life passages from Scripture that had been recited at our wedding.

First Corinthians, chapter 13, says, "If I have a faith that can move mountains, but do not have love, I am nothing . . . if I give over my body to hardship that I may boast, but do not have love, I gain nothing . . . [Love] always protects, always trusts, always hopes, always perseveres. Love never fails."

The past 2,181 miles had consummated the vows Brew and I had made to one another. We had found a way to love one another for richer and for poorer, in sickness and in health, in good times and in bad. It was clear that my husband had been the stalwart in our relationship out here and a true example of unselfishness. But there was no quantifying how much I respected him in return. I had never felt more in love with my husband than I did on top of Springer Mountain.

I did not want to leave.

Even when our friends started walking downhill to begin their long car rides home, I still had no desire to move. For one thing, I never wanted this feeling to end. I was dirty, smelly, and exhausted, but I was also more in love and at peace than I had ever been. Also, I was not sure I had the strength to make it a mile back down the mountain to the parking lot.

This is what it was *supposed* to feel like. This was one-hundred percent.

COMING DOWN THE MOUNTAIN

AUGUST 2011—THE PRESENT

The weeks that passed after Brew and I set the record were a blur. I can remember only bits and pieces of our post-trail experience, and even those memories are wrapped in a mental haze. It is hard to remember clearly what takes place when you are recovering from such an all-consuming endeavor.

The first few days after the hike, it felt as if I had just undergone a major surgery. I did not want to leave the bed, and when I did it was only to move to the couch or the hammock. I slept thirty-two of the first forty-eight hours that I spent off the trail. I didn't even have the energy to read or talk on the phone. Then came the media requests, which were surreal and sometimes frustrating.

There were reporters who chastised me or even decided not to interview me when I didn't immediately return their calls. Then there were the writers I actually spoke with, who simply printed the numbers even after I tried to give them a more holistic view of our journey.

No one seemed interested in what I'd learned or what the most valuable part of the experience had been. Instead, everyone wanted to talk about how I averaged 46.93 miles per day, or managed to consume 6,000 calories per day. They asked me if I was scared to see thirty-six bears this summer. Scared? Not at all. That was one of the highlights of the trip!

Why didn't anyone ask about the notions of living in the present or choosing something purposeful and fulfilling over something fun and easy? What about the necessity of asking other people for help and of not succumbing to the fear of failure? Or the idea that persistence and consistency can be more valuable than speed and strength? Why didn't they ask about everyone else who had helped us? Wasn't it clear that this was a group endeavor? And what about Brew? Why did no one realize that the most miraculous part of the summer was not the record, but how well my husband had loved me?!

Many of the media outlets told the story of our record without ever touching on the most important parts of the journey. Perhaps the lessons of this past summer were so counter-cultural that reporters didn't think to ask the right questions. At least the misrepresentation made it easier to disconnect from the feedback.

Opinions about our hike started to appear on websites and in my inbox, and were occasionally broadcast through the radio. The responses we heard ranged from those who questioned our record because they didn't believe I could physically cover the 2,181-mile Appalachian Trail in forty-six days, to those who decided it was really rather underwhelming, and that given the chance, most people without a full backpack could do the same thing. Just as dangerous and misinformed, but far more pleasant, were the people who thought we could do no wrong.

I think I was relatively unaffected by both the criticism and the praise. Having Brew by my side helped me to value what we had accomplished and hold on to the truth. Anyway, widespread attention is fleeting, and for the most part, I slept through our fifteen minutes of fame.

There was one incident that happened our first week off the trail, though, that I remember with striking clarity. Beyond my husband, the man I had thought about more than anyone else in recent weeks was Andrew Thompson. I went back and forth between being completely in awe of him for being such an amazing athlete and despising him for the exact same reason. But the last thing I wanted to do was talk to him.

I now knew how meaningful the overall record could be, and how difficult it was to achieve. As much as I embraced our accomplishment, I wished that it could be shared with Andrew and the other record setters of the past. I would never have been successful without studying their approaches and learning from their separate attempts. It was clear to me that a record holder never really stands alone, but rather climbs on the shoulders of the ones who have gone before him—or her.

I dreaded the call or email that I would receive from always-gracious Andrew, congratulating me on my record. I was sure he would feel compelled to say things that he didn't wholeheartedly mean. I had just taken something away from one of my heroes—how could this not be awkward?

The fateful day came when I saw his name pop up in my inbox. I did not want to click on the message, but the smiley face in the subject line encouraged me to just get it over with. When I opened the text, it contained just two words:

You bitch . . . Followed by another smiley face.

I laughed so hard that I started to cry. It was the most physical exertion I'd had since leaving Springer. I had never in my life been so proud to be called that name. Andrew had given me the most honest compliment imaginable. I knew right then that things would never be awkward between us.

I was fortunate that I could focus on rest and recovery and ease back into my work schedule because the physical effects of the trail remained for months. The initial symptoms were consuming fatigue and a decrease in appetite. I had lost about twelve pounds on the trail, but I lost another three or four the week after I finished. My metabolism was still raging but my stomach and my mind refused to eat as much as they had on the trail. I was transitioning from eating for survival to eating for enjoyment.

The next major phase of recovery was marked by dizziness and brief blackouts. I could not stand up without my head spinning, or my vision momentarily clouding over in a dark veil. I learned that I needed about ten full seconds to successfully transition from sitting to walking without passing out.

I didn't want to go to a doctor because I was convinced that I was improving, and I was scared that I might discover I'd sustained some major damage somewhere. Instead, I researched online and self-diagnosed my condition as athlete's heart. It not only explained my chest pains on the trail, but it also provided an explanation for my dizziness. According to numerous Web searches, athlete's heart is caused when the heart expands and strengthens.

The heart is a muscle, and like other muscles, it can grow. This increase in volume can cause an ache in the chest. It can also cause light-headedness because a larger chamber takes longer to fill with blood when there are sudden vertical changes.

In other words, I was like the Grinch. In the end, my experience had literally given me a bigger heart.

The calluses, blisters, and corns on my feet took about three months to harden, then peel off. At times, I picked off purple, silver-dollar-sized scales from my feet. They were dense, stiff, and always a different shape. I asked Brew if he thought we should keep a few as mementos, but he said no.

It took a long time before I had any desire to run or participate in prolonged exercise, but it was just a few weeks after I finished that my heart longed for the trail. I started by taking short two- or three-mile hikes. In direct contrast to my record hike, I enjoyed traveling down the trail at a mile and a half per hour and taking as many seated breaks as I wanted along the way.

I think my biggest regret leaving Springer Mountain was worrying about any damaged relationships that I had left along the trail. But if anything, the journey had strengthened old friendships and kindled new ones. It even brought my family together in a manner that I had always dreamed of.

Once I started hiking again, I was able to enjoy short jaunts with some of the friends who had helped me over the summer. In particular, I spent time with Melissa and Warren. It was amazing how during the record hike the A.T. had seemed to strain our relationships. Yet now, spending time together on the worn dirt path quickly healed the hurt feelings.

I was thankful that all my apologies on the trail, in person, and over the phone went so well. I was especially awed by Warren's reciprocal regret. He had never meant to make the hike more difficult for me. We talked at length about Mount Washington, about our misperceptions and misunderstandings. It only took four miles for me to realize that our time this summer hadn't fractured our connection; it had brought us closer together.

Also, for the first time in eight years, I felt like my family finally understood why I went into the woods. My oldest brother seemed proud of me in a way that I hadn't experienced before. I'd grown closer to James and Lindsay—and even more infatuated with my niece. In fact, I'd made plans to take her on her first section hike before she turned two. My dad was beaming with pride—as always. And my mom, well, my mom was there.

When I asked her if she was glad that she had come, she replied, "No. I thought your husband needed to be hospitalized because of the poison ivy on the back of his leg. And you were barely coherent. I have never been so worried about you two in my life." Translation: she wouldn't have missed it for the world.

I think if I'd expected this hike to change my life, then I would have been sorely disappointed. After a few months, everything felt pretty ordinary. Brew and I had the same friends, the same jobs, and our bank accounts had not increased. But what I had expected was that the path would change *me*—and it had.

Someone once asked me if the record was more of a physical, mental, or spiritual challenge. When I thought about it, I couldn't decide. In the end, I think it must be summed up as a love story. Not just a love story between a husband and wife, but one with multiple dimensions.

I love God and I felt called to the trail by him. I wanted to follow his voice and praise him with the talents and the gifts that he had given me.

I also love the trail. Out of all the paths that I have traveled, the Appalachian Trail remains the closest to my heart. That thin strip of dirt winding through those ancient peaks had taught me more than any other footpath and had truly changed my life. Because of that, I will always remain devoted to it and entranced by it.

And I love my husband. When I didn't have the internal drive to continue putting one foot in front of the other, I thought about all the sacrifices he was making for me. I reminded myself that he was getting only five or six hours of sleep at night, and that his days were even more emotionally demanding than my own. I know that I could not have been successful without the knowledge that he would always be at the next road crossing waiting for me.

Perhaps the most important take-away from this past summer is the realization that love is more than a feeling. True love is very different from what is often portrayed in the movies and by the media. In fact, Hollywood has really done a disservice to our perception of love. That is probably one reason why there is so much discontent and divorce in our society. It could also be why seventy-five percent of thru-hikers don't successfully complete the Appalachian Trail. Our ideas of devotion and romance are totally skewed.

True love isn't an emotion; it's a commitment—and it will be confronted by many trials and tribulations. Like the trail, love is not always easy and it is not always fun. If you really care about something or someone, you will be willing to go through hell for it (or him or her). It takes tough love for you to become your best self.

A few months before I started the trail, Brew had given me a silver necklace with a small medallion that had the word "Love" inscribed on it. I wore that necklace for half of the trail until it became so black and grimy that it started to cause a rash around my neck. Sometimes when I was struggling up a mountain or walking through a thunderstorm, I would reach for my necklace and just hold it for a minute.

When I finished the trail, I borrowed some silver polish from our neighbor and started cleaning off my necklace. I almost didn't want to. The filth told our story much better than the shining silver ever would. I decided that love should be worn. It should be worn so that others can see it, and it should be worn in the sense that it should show its age—and its miles. Love is an unending trail; and more often than not, it will *not* be pretty. It will be dirty and sticky, and it may even cause a rash (hopefully one that will go away with time or a prescription).

Some days, when I am working at home or driving down the road, I will reach for my necklace and hold it between my fingers. Immediately, I think about the hundred-degree heat and the sleet storm on Franconia Ridge. I think about shin splints and diarrhea or how Brew refused to let me quit at the base of Pico Peak. I think about how some of my best friends got on my last nerve—and what a complete diva I was in return. I reminisce about hiking behind Dutch or trying to catch up with Rambler or sharing smiles and stories with Rebekah, Matt, and Carl. I remember my nine-month-old niece clapping for me at the road crossings. I thank God once again that my flashlight didn't go out on my climb up Mount Washington and that I ran into Adam and Kadra at my absolute lowest point. I think about all of our family and friends who met us at the end, and about Brew's expression when I laid eyes on him in the Springer Mountain parking lot.

When I let go of my necklace and let it fall to my chest, next to my heart, my focus returns to my work and to my ordinary, everyday surroundings. But sometimes, in the silence that ensues, I will hear the wind through the trees or the birds warbling nearby. Then I will sense a slight twinge in my stomach and a warmth in my chest. And when I lift my eyes and gaze out the window at the mountains that surround our home in Asheville, they somehow seem closer.

In those moments, I find myself waiting, wondering, and listening. For the familiar voice that will summon me . . . when I am called again.

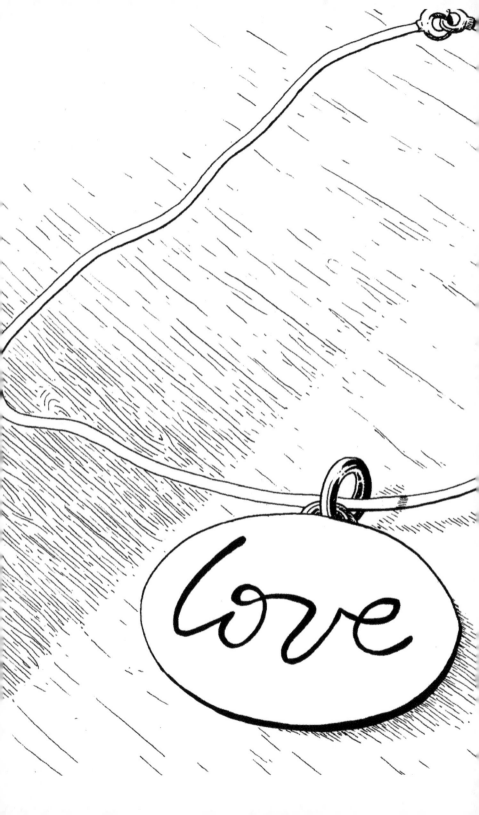

2011 ITINERARY

DAY 0   Mount Katahdin to Jo-Mary Rd—56.0 miles

DAY 1   Jo-Mary Rd to Long Pond Stream—44.2 miles

DAY 2   Long Pond Stream to Boise-Cascade Rd—45.7 miles

DAY 3   Boise-Cascade Rd to Maine 27—41.9 miles

DAY 4   Maine 27 to Houghton Fire Rd—41.0 miles

DAY 5   Houghton Fire Rd to Grafton Notch—37.9 miles

DAY 6   Grafton Notch to US 2—31.1 miles

DAY 7   US 2 to Mt. Washington—34.6 miles

DAY 8   Mt. Washington to Gale River Trail—27.8 miles

DAY 9   Gale River Trail to NH 25—38.2 miles

DAY 10   NH 25 to NH 120—42.6 miles

DAY 11   NH 120 to Stony Brook Rd—36.3 miles

DAY 12   Stony Brook Rd to Danby-Landgrove Rd—42.5 miles

DAY 13   Danby-Landgrove Rd to near Kid Gore Shelter—
43.9 miles

DAY 14   Near Kid Gore Shelter to Cheshire, MA—47.3 miles

DAY 15   Cheshire, MA to Mass. 23—48.3 miles

DAY 16   Mass. 23 to West Cornwall Rd—47.3 miles

DAY 17   West Cornwall Rd to NY 52—49.0 miles

DAY 18   NY 52 to Arden Valley Rd—49.3 miles

DAY 19   Arden Valley Rd to County 519—45.0 miles

Day 20   County 519 to PA 191—52.7 miles

DAY 21   PA 191 to past Fort Franklin Rd—48.0 miles

DAY 22   Past Fort Franklin Rd to PA 645—46.9 miles

DAY 23   PA 645 to PA 850—53.9 miles

DAY 24   PA 850 to Sandy Sod Junction—51.6 miles

DAY 25   Sandy Sod Junction to Gathland State Park—52.9 miles

DAY 26   Gathland State Park to Dicks Dome Shelter—48.7 miles

DAY 27   Dicks Dome Shelter to Skyland Service Rd—52.4 miles

DAY 28   Skyland Service Rd to Browns Gap—46.8 miles

DAY 29   Browns Gap to VA 56—52.6 miles

DAY 30   VA 56 to Matts Creek Shelter—46.9 miles

DAY 31   Matts Creek Shelter to VA 652—52.6 miles

DAY 32   VA 652 to Sinking Creek Mountain—46.9 miles

DAY 33   Sinking Creek Mountain to US 460—47.3 miles

DAY 34   US 460 to VA 615—50.3 miles

DAY 35   VA 615 to VA 16—49.2 miles

DAY 36   VA 16 to US 58—46.9 miles

DAY 37   US 58 to Vandeventer Shelter—49.8 miles

DAY 38   Vandeventer Shelter to past Doll Flats—46.1 miles

DAY 39   Past Doll Flats to the Nolichucky River—45.5 miles

DAY 40   The Nolichucky River to Camp Creek Bald—45.5 miles

DAY 41   Camp Creek Bald to Snowbird Mt.—51.3 miles

DAY 42   Snowbird Mt. to Clingmans Dome—46.3 miles

DAY 43   Clingmans Dome to NC 143—48.2 miles

DAY 44   NC 143 to Mooney Gap—52.2 miles

DAY 45   Mooney Gap to Testanee Gap—60.2 miles

DAY 46   Testanee Gap to Springer Mt.—36.2 miles

ACKNOWLEDGEMENTS

This is the story of a trail that serves as an agent of change and a metaphor for life. I am grateful for the hard work and diligence of the governing bodies that oversee the Appalachian Trail including the NPS and the ATC. I am especially appreciative of the regional trail clubs and volunteers who represent the soul of the A.T. community.

To the aptly named Pit Crew, which includes every single person who helped me down the trail in 2011, thank you for betting on the dark horse and proving that what seems impossible might just be exceptionally difficult. I wish that I could have included every person who hiked with me, prayed for me, and provided food or refuge during this journey within this book. Actually, I tried, but my editor wouldn't let me. Just know, I am able to tell a good story because you were a part of the experience.

To my family and friends who have supported me, prodded me, and believed in me even when I didn't believe in myself, thank you. James, no one else could have turned my memories into illustrations the way that you did. Thank you. Brew, being with you has made me a much better version of me. None of this would have been possible without you. I love you way more than I love the trail—and that is A LOT!

To my publishing team at Beaufort Books, thank you for helping me turn a life-changing journey into a book that is both authentic and compelling. Eric, thank you for recognizing my talent and always believing in me. Margot, thank you for making me a better writer; it has been a delight and privilege to work with you. Megan and Cindy your "legwork" getting this book to press and to the public has been invaluable. Thank you.

I look forward to having the opportunity to thank each one of you, and many others, in person . . . a little farther down the trail.